Mental Health Services in the Global Village

Edited by
LOUIS APPLEBY
RICARDO ARAYA

Mental Health Services in the Global Village

GASKELL

©The Royal College of Psychiatrists 1991

ISBN 0 902241 40 0

Gaskell is an imprint of the Royal College of Psychiatrists,
17 Belgrave Square, London SW1

Distributed in North America
by American Psychiatric Press, Inc.
ISBN 0 88048 607 4

British Library Cataloguing in Publication Data

Mental health services in the global village.
I. Appleby, Louis   II. Araya, Ricardo
362.20425

ISBN 0-902241-40-0

Cover photography Dave Jago, Sarah Robinson

Phototypeset by Dobbie Typesetting Limited, Tavistock, Devon
Printed in Great Britain

Contents

Part V. South and Central America

Part VI. International lessons

Contributors

Dr Fahad Saud Alyahya, Senior Registrar, Division of Psychiatry, Armed Forces Hospital, Riyadh, Saudi Arabia

Dr Louis Appleby, Senior Lecturer, Department of Psychiatry, University Hospital of South Manchester, Manchester, UK

Dr Ricardo Araya, Senior Registrar, Maudsley Hospital, Denmark Hill, London, UK

Dr Roberto Araya, Consultant, Hospital Psiquiatrico, Santiago, Chile

Dr Tomas Blanes, Registrar, Maudsley Hospital, Denmark Hill, London, UK

Dr Carlo Bologna, Aiuto MD, Servizio Psichiatrico USL 27, Via dello Scalo 23, 40100 Bologna, Italy

Dr Omar E. Dihoud, The Somali Counselling Project, South Bank House, London, UK

Dr Enric Duran, Research Fellow, London School of Hygiene and Tropical Medicine, Keppel Street, London, UK

Dr Ali M. El Roey, Assistant Professor in Psychiatry, Al Arab Medical University, Benghazi, Libya

Dr Eyad El-Sarraj, Gaza Community Mental Health Programme, PO Box 1049, Gaza

Dr Eduardo Iacoponi, Registrar, Maudsley Hospital, Denmark Hill, London, UK

Dr Ronaldo Ramos Laranjeira, Research Associate, Addiction Research Unit, Institute of Psychiatry, De Crespigny Park, London, UK

Dr Nasser Loza, Consultant Psychiatrist, Behman Hospital, Helwan, Cairo, Egypt

Dr Farej M. Mahdawi, Clinical Associate, Institute of Psychiatry, De Crespigny Park, London, UK

Dr Jair de Jesus Mari, Senior Lecturer, Department of Psychiatry, Escola Paulista De Medicina, São Paulo, Brazil

Dr Rodrigo Munoz-Tamayo, Child Psychiatrist, Department of Psychiatry, Hospital Militar Central, Bogotá, Colombia

Dr Iman Nabil, Registrar, Behman Hospital, Helwan, Cairo, Egypt

Dr Sekai Nhiwatiwa, Senior House Officer, Whittingham Hospital, Whittingham, Nr Preston, UK

Dr Fernan Orjuela-Mancera, Liaison Psychiatrist, Mental Health Unit, Medical Clinics Department, Clinica San Pedro Claver UP-03, Instituto de los Seguros Sociales, Bogotá, Colombia

Dr Anthony J. Pelosi, Lecturer, University Department of Psychiatry, Royal Edinburgh Hospital, Edinburgh, UK

Dr Salomon Pustilnik, Head of Child Psychiatry Department, Hospital Infantil de México, Homero 1804-804-B, Colonia Polanco, México 11550, DF

Dr Rajini Ramana, Senior Registrar, Maudsley Hospital, Denmark Hill, London, UK

Dr David Resnikoff, Consultant Psychiatrist, American British Cowdray Hospital, México DF, Insurgentes Sur 594-402, Colonia del Valle, México 03100, DF

Rowena Resnikoff, Psychiatric Nurse, Mexico City, Mexico

Dr Chiara Samele, Research Worker, Department of Psychiatry, Institute of Psychiatry, De Crespigny Park, London, UK

Dr Shekhar Saxena, Department of Psychiatry, The All India Institute of Medical Sciences, Ansari Nagar, New Delhi, India

Dr Jung Im Shim, Head of Psychiatric Department, Forensic Psychiatric Institute, Ministry of Justice Department of Psychiatric Assessment, Kong Ju, Ban Po, Korea

Dr Alisa Wacharasindhu, Department of Psychiatry, Chulalongkorn Hospital, Rama IV Road, Bangkok, Thailand

Introduction

LOUIS APPLEBY and RICARDO ARAYA

The impact of culture on mental illness is seen not only in the culture-bound syndromes or the content of delusions but also in how societies treat their mentally ill. Religion, race, tradition and politics – some of the countless competing influences on mental health provision – are themselves subject to continuous change. Variation in health care between countries may also arise because of climate, population density, the urban–rural divide, topography and sheer size. Some differences come from conquests or wars, others grow out of past mistakes.

It was to explore how the culture and contours of a country shaped its mental health services that a series of seminars was run at the Institute of Psychiatry in 1987, a series repeated annually since then. The presenters have been some of the 20–30 doctors who arrive at the Institute every year for postgraduate training, each from the sort of professional background to which few British psychiatrists are ever exposed. The seminars have provided a rare chance to compare mental health care around the world – its cultural context, its place in general health care, its obstacles and opportunities. One of the editors of this book organised the course, the other was the first presenter. Dr Doris Hollander, formerly with the World Health Organization in Zimbabwe, provided enthusiastic supervision.

It was soon clear that the information discussed would be of interest to anyone who valued first-hand accounts of how psychiatry is practised in other countries. It seemed logical then to convert the series into a short book and, conveniently, Gaskell had already published a near-predecessor which could be expanded and updated, *Psychiatry in Developing Countries*, edited by Stephen Brown.

But which countries to include? The chapters here cover all the world's regions. Developed as well as developing countries are represented, as are countries in transition, such as Thailand and Brazil. Mexico is a land of massive urban influx; Saudi Arabia a land of massive wealth. India is largely rural but infinitely varied; Egypt largely desert but also metropolitan: both have powerful ancient traditions. How do these varying features affect health care?

Some of those selected illustrate mental services in a changing welfare ideology – Italy and Britain are examples. For many – Chile, Spain, Zimbabwe and Korea – the treatment of the mentally ill is a direct product of their recent political past. Others, such as Colombia and Libya, are countries whose image abroad normally leaves little room for mention of health.

Two chapters are different, presenting not a country but a population without a country. One describes Somali refugees in neighbouring Ethiopia and in the foreign landscape of East London, and was written as the long-standing civil war in Somalia appeared to be near its climax. The second is a description of health in the occupied Palestinian territories, written before the first violence of the Gulf War.

The authors are not the leading academics or administrators of their countries, at least not yet. That is their strength. They are junior enough to have worked in their countries' health services without feeling responsible for them. As editors, we have encouraged them to be provocative and opinionated, if necessary idealistic, and to use what information they could obtain (in several cases few data existed) to advocate radical change. Some may well end up in senior positions of authority where they may be able to bring about what they now propose. The American poet Robert Frost once said he never dared to be radical when young for fear of being conservative when old. We shall see.

I. Asia

1 India: quality and access are the priorities

RAJINI RAMANA and SHEKHAR SAXENA

India, a vast peninsula, comprises 2.4% of the world's land area and supports 15.5% of the world's population. It is a multilingual and multi-ethnic federal democracy which is home to 843 million people, 40% of whom are aged 14 years or less. There is no state religion: Hinduism is the most common, followed by Islam, Sikhism and Christianity. India is divided into 31 states, each with its own parliamentary government headed by a chief minister. Issues such as education and health are under state jurisdiction. The central government, which has proportional representation from the various states, handles issues like foreign policy and defence. The head of state is the president but executive power is vested in a prime minister chosen by the political party with a majority in the lower house of parliament. Governing a country that is so diverse is incredibly difficult, and long-standing inter-communal strife has made it even more so.

Population control remains a pressing problem. The birth rate is about 36 per thousand and the annual average exponential growth rate was estimated at 2.25% in the early 1980s (Park & Park, 1986). The national literacy rate is 52% for men and 25% for women although it varies from state to state. Kerala, a southern state, has the highest rate (70%) and Arunachal Pradesh in the north-east has the lowest (20%). About two-thirds of the population live in rural areas, although continuing large-scale migration to already overcrowded urban areas is changing this proportion. In general, urban areas have better amenities than rural areas, and this disproportionate distribution of services is particularly evident in health care.

Despite considerable technological advancement since independence in 1947, India remains a poor country with limited resources, a low gross national product (£163 billion in 1990), and low per capita income (£190 in 1990). However, the economy grew at an unprecedented rate of more than 5% in the 1980s, and the government estimates that 29.2% of the population now live under the poverty line, compared with 48% in the late 1970s. Facilities such as basic sanitation and clean drinking water are not available to all. However, these overall generalisations hide great

3

disparity – between different states where political and physical climates, the degree of industrialisation, unemployment rates and social conditions vary, and between different socio-economic classes in the same state. A burgeoning urban middle class and a small upper class enjoy comparatively high standards of living and there is an 8% industrial growth rate.

Structure of health care services

Three sectors provide health care in India: public, private and voluntary. Public health care services are administered independently by each state government, although the structure of service provision is uniform throughout the country. Each state is divided into administrative districts and each district is further subdivided into blocks; health care services are provided at each of these levels, as shown in Fig. 1.1. These services are free, although within the system a better standard of care can be purchased. The public health service involves the local community at the primary levels of health care and uses this resource to great advantage. Ideologically, this community health care system is among the best in the world. Unfortunately, lack of money and resources have undermined it and it functions adequately only in a few areas. Staff shortages are a major problem, particularly in rural areas.

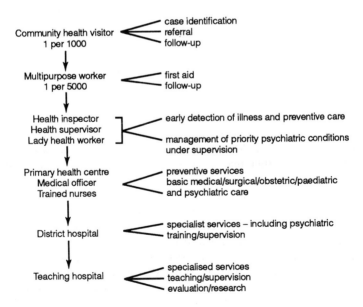

Fig. 1.1. Levels of health care in India

Parallel services offering a higher standard of care are also provided through state and central government agencies. For example, employees of private sector businesses can purchase health care by voluntary contributions to a government-managed health insurance scheme which provides a parallel system of hospitals. Also, major public sector employers like Indian Railways provide their own health services. Most of these services are confined to urban areas.

Private health care is expensive and standards vary greatly. Most cities have modern, well equipped hospitals offering specialist care. Consumer demand for better health care has fuelled a growth in the private health care sector, and private health insurance schemes are becoming more popular. Unfortunately these are almost exclusive to urban areas. Between the public and private systems there exist non-profit-making, autonomous hospitals and voluntary organisations which deliver excellent health care and charge clients according to their ability to pay.

India's major health problems are malnutrition, infectious diseases and population control. The country's annual health budget, which is about 2% of the total budget, is barely sufficient to tackle these. The shortage of trained personnel and essential supplies further compounds the problem. Given these constraints, providing adequate health care for over 800 million people over such a large area poses incredible problems. Providing appropriate and adequate care for the mentally ill has therefore, of necessity, not been a priority. Urban areas are better served than rural areas and this is best demonstrated by the difference in the infant mortality rates: 65 per thousand in urban areas compared to 114 per thousand in rural areas.

Mental health care

Mental illness has been recognised and treated in India for over 2000 years. *Ayurveda*, a complex system of traditional medicine, evolved three millennia ago and is still practised widely. There are entire sections dealing with psychological problems in *Charaka Samhita* and *Susruta Samhita*, the two ancient texts on *Ayurveda*. Some of the problems described here are clearly recognisable to the modern psychiatrist. *Unani*, an ancient form of Arabic medicine, is the other major system of traditional medicine. Both these systems are officially recognised by the government, which funds their hospitals and research institutions; indeed many modern medical institutions have departments of traditional medicine. Various other forms of indigenous medicine exist, such as those followed by the *mantrawadis*, who use astrology and charms, and the *patris*, who act as mediums for spirits and demons.

The importance of these systems of medicine in psychiatry cannot be overemphasised. Even in areas with access to modern psychiatric care, a significant number of patients are seen by traditional healers before they are seen by psychiatrists, and in some remote rural areas traditional healers are the only form of help available to the mentally ill. Studies have shown that about 60% of patients first see a traditional healer (Kapur, 1975; Sethi, 1979). These practitioners often have a much wider social function than that of a healer and exert great influence on local attitudes to health care, especially in rural areas. It is, therefore, often essential for modern health workers to enlist their support and to collaborate with them. The methods of treatment employed by these practitioners vary. Medicinal herbs such as *rauwolfia*, special diets and simple behavioural treatments have been used for centuries by the Ayurvedic physicians. Some offer valuable supportive psychotherapy and help rehabilitate patients. However, others use dangerous methods such as treatment with mercury-containing compounds and arsenic. Treatment methods such as chaining and beating the evil spirits out of the body are practised by some but are becoming more uncommon. One of the main remits of the National Mental Health Programme set up by the central government in 1982 is to educate people about mental illness and to eradicate these brutal forms of treatment.

Another important cultural feature is the structure of the family. Traditionally, India has had an extended family system in which the sons of each couple and their families lived under the same roof, with three generations often living together. This system provided valuable economic and emotional support to family members, and could accommodate disabled members with ease. However, it was sometimes detrimental as patients could be isolated within the family and denied access to proper medical care. The extended family system is on the decline in urban areas due to recent socio-political changes. Nuclear families are more common in the urban areas and they face the same problems as a nuclear family in a Western country when required to care for a mentally ill member.

The International Pilot Study of Schizophrenia (World Health Organization, 1979) found the outcome of schizophrenia was substantially better in Indian than in European and North American centres. This was attributed to tolerant family attitudes to illness and handicap, given the association between poor outcome in schizophrenia and high expressed emotion (EE) (Brown *et al*, 1972; Vaughn & Leff, 1976). The finding spawned extensive research into differences in EE between developed countries in the West and India (Wig *et al*, 1987a; Wig *et al*, 1987b; Leff *et al*, 1987). The relationship between high EE and poor outcome appears to be the same as in Anglo-American cultures. Indian relatives were found to express fewer positive remarks, fewer critical comments and less over-involvement than their Western counterparts. Relatives in rural areas were found to be less expressive than those in urban areas, but this difference did not lead to a significant difference in outcome between these areas. Various explanations have been put forward for the differences in 'emotional interaction' between these cultures and their effect on the course and outcome of schizophrenia. However, it is open to debate whether the rating of EE can be done cross-culturally using the Camberwell Family Interview (Brown & Rutter, 1966), an instrument designed for use in a Western culture, and whether this difference in levels of EE can adequately explain the difference in outcome.

Prevalence of mental illness

It is only since independence and in the last three decades that studies have been carried out to collect epidemiological data on mental illness in India (Table 1.1). Some of these studies are methodologically flawed and since screening procedures and diagnostic categories varied in the earlier studies, the rates may not be strictly comparable. However, they demonstrated that mental illness is prevalent in India and wiped out the colonial belief that mental illness is not a problem of predominantly agrarian developing countries. They also provided a database for national planning of services. The National Mental Health Programme (1982) has estimated from available data that the point prevalence of serious mental illness is 10–20 per thousand, and that of neuroses and psychosomatic disorders is 20–40 per thousand. Thus, a staggering 20–30 million adults are in need of psychiatric services

TABLE 1.1
Epidemiological surveys on mental illness

Study	Population studied	Prevalence rate per 1000 of all psychiatric disorders
Surya *et al*, 1964	urban, Pondicherry	9.5
Dube, 1970	rural, semi-rural and urban	17.99
Elnagar *et al*, 1971	rural	27
Sethi *et al*, 1972	rural	39
Verghese *et al*, 1973	urban	66.5
Nandi *et al*, 1975	rural	102
Carstairs & Kapur, 1976	rural	369
ICMR Collaborative Study, 1980	urban	
	Bangalore	11.1
	Baroda	4.6
	Calcutta	8.3
	Patiala	14.1

With only 2000 trained psychiatrists and fewer than 1000 psychiatric nurses, there is a massive shortfall in service provision. There is little information on the number of children in need of psychiatric services, and often no provisions are made to supply a service for them. The working party for the National Mental Health Programme estimated that existing services are able to provide adequate care for only 10% of those who need it. There is clearly a need for more high-quality research on the prevalence of various disorders, particularly the differences between various ethnic and socioeconomic groups. However, research of this kind is expensive and time-consuming. With major limitations in budgets and personnel, priority has rightfully been given to research into improving the quality and availability of appropriate mental health care.

Existing services

Psychiatric care can be obtained through public mental hospitals and psychiatric units in general hospitals, as well as through the private and voluntary sectors. Before independence, psychiatric care was only available in large mental hospitals modelled on the European asylums of that age, which provided custodial care. The best of these were located in hill-stations such as Ranchi and treated only Europeans. Currently, there are 42 public sector mental hospitals with a total of 20 000 beds, half of which are occupied by chronic patients. Admissions and discharges are governed by the antiquated Indian Lunacy Act of 1912, and every admission involves a lengthy bureaucratic procedure which often greatly delays appropriate treatment. While these hospitals leave much to be desired, they are necessary for the more severely disabled patients. The government is attempting to improve conditions by linking the hospitals with university departments of psychiatry.

Virtually no care was available outside mental hospitals until 1933 when Girendra Bose opened the first general hospital psychiatric unit in Calcutta (Wig, 1978), long before the term 'liaison psychiatry' was coined. After independence, and especially in the 1960s and '70s, the number of these units grew rapidly and many of the medical schools in India now have psychiatric units. Unlike their counterparts in the West, these units often provide the only psychiatric service for the area and are frequently understaffed and overcrowded. They are a vast improvement on the old mental hospitals as they are more acceptable and accessible to the local community, and admissions are not governed by the Indian Lunacy Act of 1912. These general hospital psychiatric units have been primarily responsible for making psychiatry more acceptable as a career as they became actively involved in mainstream undergraduate medical education and in hospital services. More importantly, they have been instrumental in lessening the social stigma attached to mental illness, although this stigma has by no means been eradicated.

Private psychiatric services are available in most cities and are expanding rapidly, depriving an already starved state of much-needed medical manpower. The impact that these services have had on the quality and availability of mental health care has not been investigated.

The voluntary sector provides a valuable source of quality care. The services provided include rehabilitative and supportive care, residential facilities and family support. Private medical schools like the one at Vellore in south India have psychiatric units providing excellent care, and specialist training and research facilities. However, the services provided by the voluntary sector cannot be expected to make up for deficiencies in state-run facilities.

Child psychiatry clinics, also called child guidance clinics, are run by most teaching-hospital psychiatry units and, in some places, by psychologists.

However, in-patient facilities are extremely limited and the service provided is grossly inadequate; these facilities also have to cater for the needs of the 7.5 million mentally retarded children in India. Plans to integrate child psychiatric services into the existing child health services have been hampered by the sheer magnitude of other more pressing child health problems. Most of the inadequate existing services were developed after 1960 and nearly all are concentrated in cities. Treatment and rehabilitative services for this group are minimal and need to be vastly improved (Bartlett, 1987).

Service provision for the addictions has increased substantially in the last five years in response to the increase in the problem in the 1980s. The government has provided funds for developing six regional centres, and numerous voluntary and self-help agencies have also been established. Again, most of these are in large cities and this leaves other areas relatively underserved (Mohan *et al*, 1981). There are no official forensic psychiatric services, although separate enclosures for forensic patients exist in some hospitals. The central government is still debating the introduction of a new mental health act – guidelines for which were drafted almost ten years ago.

Indian psychiatrists have actively involved the family in the care of the patient since the 1960s (Kohlmeyer & Fernandez, 1963). In some in-patient units with insufficient nursing support, family members often fulfil this role. In Vellore, the family is admitted along with the patient, in separate housing units, and they are closely involved in the treatment programme (Chacko, 1967). It has been shown that involving the family to this extent reduced the admission period by up to 75% and improved treatment compliance (Narayan *et al*, 1972; Narayan, 1977; Bhatti *et al*, 1980). Needless to say, this particular approach is feasible in only a few situations and may become increasingly difficult as families are often nuclear with both parents employed. The better outcome of schizophrenia reported in India (Cooper & Sartorius, 1977; World Health Organization, 1979) compared to the West may be related both to the acceptance of the patient by the family and society and to the support given to patients by the family. Thus, the family often fulfils the role taken by rehabilitation services in the West. Unfortunately, this role of the family has been taken for granted and rehabilitation and aftercare services are almost non-existent; this is potentially a major problem in urban areas with an increasing number of nuclear families.

Availability and training of personnel

There are currently about 2000 psychiatrists in India, most of whom are locally trained. It is estimated that there are fewer than 1000 each of trained clinical psychologists, psychiatric nurses and psychiatric social workers. Psychiatry is part of the undergraduate medical curriculum, but only 50% of medical schools have departments of psychiatry and this is a handicap to adequate training. Only 25% of medical schools offer postgraduate training in psychiatry; about 150 psychiatrists are trained every year.

Training of other personnel is usually possible only in specialised academic centres.

Thus the major constraint that India faces, in common with other developing countries, is the extreme shortage of trained personnel. The quickest, and probably the most effective, way of enhancing the availability of mental health manpower in developing countries faced with this situation, is to train and use non-specialised health workers at the primary care level (World Health Organization, 1975; Giel & Harding, 1976). This approach is particularly attractive because the care provided by these workers is likely to be more acceptable to the community. The Raipur Rani trial (Wig *et al*, 1981) demonstrated that community health workers (CHWs) were able to acquire the skills to diagnose, and to an extent treat, common psychiatric problems using a limited range of inexpensive drugs. A group in Bangalore, South India, reached similar conclusions (Isaac *et al*, 1982; Chandrasekhar *et al*, 1981). Harding *et al* (1980) have shown, in a four-centre study, that primary health staff can correctly identify about one-third of the psychiatric morbidity occurring at the primary care level. Most of the morbidity was of the 'neurotic' type that one would expect to see in a general practitioner's surgery in the UK; about one-third to two-thirds of psychiatric morbidity is missed at this level worldwide (Goldberg & Blackwell, 1970; Giel & Le Nobel, 1971). Thus, using primary level workers and despecialising mental health care seems to be the best option for India to follow in the 1990s. Training programmes and manuals designed for these workers have been developed in collaboration with the World Health Organization (WHO) and used successfully (Srinivasa Murthy & Wig, 1983).

Proposed services

The National Mental Health Programme was formulated by an expert working party in collaboration with the WHO and along the guidelines set out by the WHO expert committee (1975). The programme was officially adopted by the government in 1982 as its policy on mental health, but it has yet to be implemented in full. The main objectives of the programme are as follows:

(a) to adopt the plan in all states within one year and to work out, with the help of a task force and a multidisciplinary national co-ordinating group, a training programme for health workers

(b) to train within five years at least 5000 non-medical professionals and at least 20% of doctors working in primary health centres (PHCs, see Fig. 1.1) to detect and manage priority psychiatric problems

(c) to create the post of district psychiatrist in at least 50% of administrative districts within five years, to provide specialist care and supervise and educate primary care personnel

(d) to provide psychiatric units with in-patient beds in all medical college hospitals within five years

(e) to enable each state to provide additional support and facilities for the training of mental health care professionals within five years
(f) to appoint a programme officer in each state to organise and supervise the programme, and provide the focal point for the gathering of evaluative data.

This plan seems to provide an answer to the most pressing problem: the delivery of adequate primary mental health care despite an extreme shortage of personnel. However, it has yet to be implemented fully in most states, seven years after its adoption.

Recommendations

The major mental health care priority in India is to improve the availability and quality of services; the major constraints are grossly inadequate finance and manpower. When pressing problems like malnutrition and infectious diseases still have to be tackled, it is unlikely that mental health care will receive a substantially increased share of the health budget in the foreseeable future. The shortage of trained professionals is more serious. Plans for training personnel have been carefully thought out and special training programmes for primary care personnel have been successfully used (Srinivasa Murthy & Wig, 1983). However, none of these can be implemented if a career in the health services is not an attractive proposition. Government salaries cannot compare with those in the private sector and it is unrealistic to expect people to work in rural areas for a less than attractive salary. If the state needs manpower, it must offer financial and other incentives to attract suitable persons, in the same way that it enables the defence services to offer special incentives. There must also be a concerted effort to improve the professional status of nursing, social work and psychology in order to make these careers that school-leavers will seriously consider.

While the National Mental Health Programme is carefully considered overall, certain aspects require more attention. Most of the planned services may in fact be appropriate only for adults: provision for child psychiatric services is woefully inadequate, and specific action to overcome this must be made part of the programme. There is little existing collaboration with non-medical agencies, especially schoolteachers, the police and non-medical community agencies, and no plans have been made to ensure their involvement in the future. The rights of the mentally ill receive scant mention. The lay public needs to be educated about their rights when mentally ill, and the proposed new mental health act must be discussed publicly and implemented soon in order to protect these rights. Although this may not appear to be a current priority, a programme that aims to address mental health needs through the next decade of rapid socio-economic change must take mental health legislation more seriously.

Another aspect of mental health care that has been inadequately dealt with is the availability of drugs. It is not uncommon to see representatives from multinational drug companies promoting their latest product, despite the fact that a day's dosage often costs more than the patient's monthly income. It is the responsibility of the state to ensure that essential drugs are consistently available and to take measures to reduce cost by legislating for local manufacture and bulk purchase. Action should be considered to reduce the private sector resources currently used to manufacture profitable but non-essential drugs and increase production of essential drugs.

The National Mental Health Programme rightly stresses the need for appropriate research, especially in the areas of service delivery and evaluation. Issues such as the development of appropriate measurement scales, service needs and delivery, and training needs and methods must be focused on in the immediate future. However the balance between service and research is a changing one; constant re-evaluation will be necessary to ensure that well directed research helps to close the gap between needs and resources as Indian mental health care services continue to evolve into the next decade.

References

BARTLETT, L. B. (1987) Child psychiatric services in India. *Bulletin of the Royal College of Psychiatrists*, **11**, 122.

BHATTI, R. S., JANAKIRAMAIAH, N. & CHANNABASAVANNA, S. M. (1980) Family psychiatric ward treatment in India. *Family Process*, **19**, 193.

BROWN, G. W., BIRLEY, J. L. T. & WING, J. K. (1972) Influence of family life on the course of schizophrenic disorders: a replication. *British Journal of Psychiatry*, **121**, 241–258.

BROWN, G. W. & RUTTER, M. (1966) The measurement of family activities and relationships: a methodological study. *Human Relations*, **19**, 241–263.

CARSTAIRS, G. M. & KAPUR, R. L. (1976) *The Great Universe of Kota*. London: Hogarth Press.

CHACKO, R. (1967) Family participation in the treatment and rehabilitation of the mentally ill. *Indian Journal of Psychiatry*, **9**, 328.

CHANDRASEKHAR, C. R., ISAAC, M. K., KAPUR, R. L., *et al* (1981) Management of priority mental disorders in the community. *Indian Journal of Psychiatry*, **23**, 179.

COOPER, J. & SARTORIUS, N. (1977) Cultural and temporal variations in schizophrenia – a speculation on the importance of industrialization. *British Journal of Psychiatry*, **130**, 50.

DUBE, K. C. (1970) A study of prevalence and biosocial variables in mental illness in a rural and an urban community in Uttarpradesh, India. *Acta Psychiatrica Scandinavica*, **46**, 327.

ELNAGAR, M. M., MAITRA, P. & RAO, M. M. (1971) Mental health in a rural Indian community. *British Journal of Psychiatry*, **118**, 499.

GIEL, R. & LE NOBEL, C. P. J. (1971) Neurotic instability in a Dutch village. *Acta Psychiatrica Scandinavica*, **47**, 462.

——— & HARDING, T. W. (1976) Psychiatric priorities in developing countries. *British Journal of Psychiatry*, **128**, 513–522.

GOLDBERG, D. P. & BLACKWELL, B. (1970) Psychiatric illness in general practice: a detailed study using a new method of case identification. *British Medical Journal*, *ii*, 439.

HARDING, T. W., DE ARANGO, M. V., BALTAZAR, J., *et al* (1980) Mental disorders in primary health care: a study of their frequency and diagnosis in four developing countries. *Psychological Medicine*, **10**, 231.

ISAAC, M. K., KAPUR, R. L., CHANDRASEKHAR, C. R., *et al* (1982) Mental health delivery through primary care – development and evaluation of a pilot training programme. *Indian Journal of Psychiatry*, **24**, 131–138.

KAPUR, R. L. (1975) Mental health care in rural India: a study of existing patterns and their implications for future policy. *British Journal of Psychiatry*, **127**, 286.

KOHLMEYER, W. A. & FERNANDEZ, X. (1963) Psychiatry in India: family approach in the treatment of mental disorders. *American Journal of Psychiatry*, **119**, 1033.

LEFF, J., WIG, N. N., GHOSH, A., *et al* (1987) Influence of relatives' expressed emotion on the course of schizophrenia in Chandigarh. *British Journal of Psychiatry*, **151**, 166–173.

MOHAN, D., SETHI, H. S., TONGUE, E. (eds) (1980) *Current Research in Drug Abuse in India*. New Delhi: Gemini Printers.

NANDI, D. N., AGMANY, S., GANGULY, H., *et al* (1975) Psychiatric disorders in a rural community in West Bengal – an epidemiological study. *Indian Journal of Psychiatry*, **17**, 87.

NARAYAN, H. S. (1977) Experience with group and family therapy in India. *International Journal of Group Psychotherapy*, **32**, 517.

——, EMBA, P. & REDDY, G. N. N. (1972) Review of treatment in the family ward. *Indian Journal of Psychiatry*, **14**, 123.

NATIONAL MENTAL HEALTH PROGRAMME (1982) New Delhi: Director General of Health Services.

PARK, J. E. & PARK, K. (1986) *Textbook of Preventive and Social Medicine (11th edn)*. Jabalpur, India: Banarsidas Bhanot.

SETHI, B. B. & TRIVEDI, J. K. (1979) Socioeconomic variables and manifestations of ill-health in patients who attended traditional healers' clinics. *Indian Journal of Psychiatry*, **21**, 133.

——, GUPTA, S. C., KUMER, R., *et al* (1972) Psychiatric survey of 500 rural families. *Indian Journal of Psychiatry*, **14**, 183–196.

SRINIVASA MURTHY, R. & WIG, N. N. (1983) The WHO collaborative study on strategies for extending mental health care IV: a training approach to enhancing the availability of mental health manpower in a developing country. *American Journal of Psychiatry*, **140**, 11.

SURYA, N. C., DUTTA, S. P., GOPALAKRISHNA, R., *et al* (1964) Mental morbidity in Pondicherry (1962–63). *Transactions of All India Institute of Mental Health*, **4**, 50–56.

VERGHESE, A. M., BEIG, A., SENSAMAN, L. A., *et al* (1973) A social and psychiatric study of a representative group of families in Vellore Town. *Indian Journal of Medical Research*, **61**, 808.

VAUGHN, C. & LEFF, J. P. (1976) The influence of family and social factors on the course of psychiatric illness. A comparison of schizophrenic and depressed neurotic patients. *British Journal of Psychiatry*, **129**, 125–137.

WIG, N. N. (1978) Psychiatric units in general hospitals – right time for evaluation. *Indian Journal of Psychiatry*, **20**, 1.

——, MENON, D. K., BEDI, H., *et al* (1987*a*) The cross-cultural transfer of ratings of relatives' expressed emotion. *British Journal of Psychiatry*, **151**, 156–160.

——, ——, ——, *et al* (1987*b*) Distribution of expressed emotion components among relatives of schizophrenic patients in Aarhus and Chandigarh. *British Journal of Psychiatry*, **151**, 160–165.

——, MURTHY, R. S. & HARDING, T. W. (1981) A model for rural psychiatric services: the Raipur Rani experience. *Indian Journal of Psychiatry*, **23**, 275–290.

WORLD HEALTH ORGANIZATION (1975) *Organization of mental health services in developing countries*. Technical Report Series No 564. Geneva: WHO.

—— (1979) *Schizophrenia: An International Follow-up Study, Vol II*. Chichester and New York: John Wiley.

2 Thailand: a growing service in a growing economy

ALISA WACHARASINDHU

Thailand is located in the heart of South-East Asia in an area of 513 115 km² (about the size of France). The country is divided into four regions (the North, the North-East, the Central and the South), and administratively into Bangkok Metropolis, the nation's capital in the central region, and 73 provinces. A province (*changwat*) is divided into districts (*ampoe*), subdistricts (*tambon*), and villages (*mu-ban*). There are approximately 700 districts, 500 subdistricts, and 50 000 villages.

The country has a population of approximately 55 million (1989) with about 75% of the total population living in the rural areas, and the remaining 25% clustered mainly in Bangkok and other urban areas. Bangkok has an estimated population of 6–7 million, while the second largest city, Chiang Mai, has a population of about 1.5 million. The population shows a rich ethnic diversity – Thai, Chinese, Mon, Khmer, Burmese, Malay, and Indian stock as the result of the assimilation of immigrants from neighbouring countries – with little social friction.

Buddhism is the national religion, the centre of the Thai way of life, and forms the foundation of most attitudes. Buddhist temples are the heart of social as well as religious life, especially in the rural areas where they also serve as educational institutions. However, religious freedom is guaranteed, and all major religions can be found in practice.

Thailand's governing system is a constitutional monarchy which has a democratic parliamentary form of government with the King as the Head of State, a system similar to that of the United Kingdom. Significantly, Thailand is the only South-East Asian country never to have been colonised by Western powers. This undoubtedly accounts for its unique character, continually developed during more than 700 years of independence. The monarchy remains as strong as ever and is the central, unifying element in the Thai triad of nation, religion and King. The present monarch, King Bhumibol Adulyadej, is popular because of his involvement in many developmental projects for the poor in the rural areas.

Economic and social transitions

National development for the past 30 years has followed the directions stated in the five-year National Economic and Social Development Plans. This development has resulted in a better standard of living for Thai people. The Gross National Product (GNP) increased 18-fold from 1961 to 1985, while the average annual per capita income increased about 10-fold. In the field of social development, both education and public welfare services have been upgraded and distributed more widely, and the quality of life of the Thai people has improved correspondingly. In education, for instance, there are now secondary schools in all districts in the country. In public welfare, 92 % of all districts now boast a hospital and 98 % of all subdistricts contain health centres, while primary health care services are available in no less than 90 % of all villages in the country (Office of the National Economic and Social Development Board, 1987).

Traditionally an agrarian nation, Thailand today is a country with a complex, multi-faceted economy embracing industries that employ sophisticated technology. At the same time, with its abundance and diversity of natural resources, Thailand not only maintains agricultural self-sufficiency but is also one of the largest food exporters in the world.

Thailand is in a period of transition from a basic agricultural economy to one based more on manufacturing and service industries. This transition has meant increased urbanisation and rural–urban migration with a concomitant change in the way of life of the Thai. The family structure has, for instance, changed from a large extended family to a much smaller unit. The success of the country's family planning programme has led to a reduction in the average family size from 6.4 persons in 1978 to 5.4 persons in 1987.

These changes both accentuate existing development problems and open new challenges. The existing poverty and income disparities remain. Per capita income in Bangkok is 7.2 times higher than in the North-East, an increase from a gap of 6.9 times in 1978. About 25.2 % of the population is below the poverty line, an increase from 23 % in 1981 (although the figure rose sharply to 29.5 % in 1986 due to the fall in the prices of agricultural products worldwide). Urban poverty and unemployment, especially among unskilled labourers, are other serious problems that must be dealt with.

Poverty has intensified some old problems, especially social problems such as prostitution and drugs. Prostitution thrives not only domestically but also as a labour export to various European countries and Japan. As for drugs, although Thailand is situated in the Golden Triangle where opium is the main product, the government eradication programme in co-operation with international agencies has been successful in curtailing drug production at least on the Thai border side. However, domestically, other easy-access drugs such as marijuana and solvents are becoming problems among teenagers and unskilled labourers.

In spite of years of development of basic education and health services, many problems remain. In health many challenges have to be dealt with to improve the quality of life, such as mental health problems from the stress of modern urban life, and acquired immune deficiency syndrome (AIDS), which will be discussed later.

Health service

Western medicine was introduced to Thailand 100 years ago. There are approximately 30 large hospitals in Bangkok, and in the provinces there are large general hospitals, 14 of which have been designated as regional medical centres. There are over 500 district or community hospitals and there are health stations in all subdistricts. Despite this framework, the population coverage is still poor. Too many people still become ill from preventable diseases. In addition, the narrow-based health service system and the non-existence of catchment areas allow the patients to converge on the larger hospitals, including the medical school hospitals. This situation restricts teaching and research in the medical school hospitals and creates an overlap of responsibilities for patient care. The hospitals and health stations which form the major part of the health service are under the jurisdiction of the Ministry of Public Health. The medical school hospitals are run by the Office of University Affairs. Moreover, there are many other hospitals run by other government agencies. For example, the Ministry of Defence has its own hospitals and health service centres; the Ministry of the Interior has its hospitals for the police force and their families. The Bangkok Metropolis also has hospitals and health centres in the capital. There are many private clinics and hospitals located almost everywhere in the country. The numbers and distribution of beds and health personnel are shown in Tables 2.1–2.4.

The Thai Prime Minister and the Director-General of the World Health Organization (WHO) are signatories to a health charter committing Thailand to the goal of 'Health for All' through Primary Health Care (PHC). The definition of PHC in Thailand is considered to be health care of the people, by the people and for the people, to be supported by other levels of health care and other sectors of social development.

To fill the gaps between the communities and the health service system, primary health care has relied heavily on villagers who have been briefly trained, called Village Health Communicators (VHCs) and Village Health Volunteers (VHVs). An office of PHC in the Ministry of Public Health organises the training of the VHCs and VHVs, with the intention of producing at least 10 VHCs and 1 VHV for each of the 50 000 villages. Thus the total numbers of VHCs and VHVs to be trained are 500 000 and 50 000 respectively.

TABLE 2.1
Bed provision for Bangkok Metropolis and the other provinces

Area	No. of beds	No. of population per bed
Whole country	69 049	748
Bangkok Metropolis	16 889	336
Other provinces	52 160	882

(Division of Health Statistics, 1985)

TABLE 2.2
Number of health facilities (1985)

Type of Health Institution	Number
Health Centres	7235
Community Health Centres	365
Health Centres	55
(Bureau of Health, Bangkok Metropolitan Authority)	
Private Clinics	8695

(Division of Health Statistics, 1985)

TABLE 2.3
Medical and health personnel by type of administration 1985

Category of personnel by type of administration	Physicians	Nurses[1]	Technical nurses	Auxiliary nurses	Midwives	Health workers[2]
Total	8650	28 019	10 664	22 443	7716	7343
Government	4773	21 110	10 560	17 142	6945	7316
Ministries of Public Health	4401	16 036	10 550	12 293	6931	7290
Other Ministries	2630	5462	10	4849	14	26
State enterprise	250	1958	–	1024	92	1
Municipality	363	1683	3	400	83	24
Private	1006	2880	101	3877	596	2

1. Professional Nurse, Nurse Practitioner, Nursing and Midwifery, Public Health Nurse (PHN), Anaesthetic Nurse, or Nurse Specialist.
2. Graduated from public college or equivalent.
(Division of Health Statistics, 1985)

TABLE 2.4
The ratio between population and medical and health personnel of each category in Bangkok Metropolis and other provinces in 1985

Area	No. per doctor	No. per nurse
Whole country	5978	1336
Bangkok Metropolis	1453	523
Other provinces	9706	1663

(Division of Health Statistics, 1985)

The universities have a role in recognising manpower production, research and services to fit in with the expanded and integrated health service. There are several joint activities undertaken between the universities and the Ministry of Public Health such as rural doctors' training, community medicine programmes and a health policy study centre.

The Ministry of Public Health has worked closely with the National Economic and Social Development Board, which acted as co-ordinator of the collaborative efforts among the Ministries of Education, Agriculture and the Interior. A basic minimal needs (BMN) approach (according to WHO) has also been introduced to specify the minimal needs of individuals, families and communities with regard to food and water supplies, environment, health care and education, and is used to define both goals and deficiencies in the system. Village self-management, and technical co-operation among developing villages are under way.

There are many non-government organisations. A 'folk doctor' foundation supports PHC through production of educational materials and training, and the Folk Doctor group has conducted and propagated the training of monks for PHC, the temples being great social assets in Buddhism. There are organisations dealing with family planning and other community activities. King Bhumibol Adulyadej is the country's best-loved healer, to whom numerous Thai rural poor turn for medical help. He has initiated many medical projects, both preventive and curative. He arranges to bring a team of doctors, personnel and supplies with him to the districts to give treatment to the local people free of charge. Doctors on the team come from various hospitals. He also provides basic medical supplies to temples and schools in rural areas for local use and has long been a supporter of medical and biology-related research projects.

Despite these modern health organisations, there are still those who do not have access to the health services they need. Moreover, there are others who are aware of the available facilities but still rely on traditional healers such as Buddhist monks, faith healers and dispensers of herbs and traditional medicine. Some of these are undoubtedly useful in that they can at least give psychological support but they may also be the cause of delayed diagnosis and treatment of serious disease. It is not at all uncommon for people to visit both modern health services and traditional healers: this is acceptable to most health professions.

General health indicators

The life expectancy of Thai males is 61–75 years, and of females is 67–80 years. The mortality rate is 4.2 per 1000 population (1987) and the infant mortality rate, 10.6 per 1000 live births. The five leading causes of death according to ICD-9 (World Health Organization, 1978) are diseases of the circulation and heart, disorders of the digestive system, accidents, neoplasm and respiratory disease.

The three leading causes of out-patient consultation are disorders of the respiratory system, digestive diseases, and infections. The three most common causes of in-patient treatment are delivery and complications of pregnancy, enteritis and other diarrhoeal diseases, and accidents.

AIDS is a recent threat. By the end of 1989, about one million Thai people had had blood tests for human immunodeficiency virus (HIV) status. There were 34 AIDS patients, 103 with AIDS-related complex, and 12 793 HIV-positive cases, of whom 11 082 were male and 1711 female. The two main patterns of behaviour leading to AIDS in Thailand are sexual promiscuity, both homosexual and heterosexual, mainly via prostitutes, and intravenous drug use, especially heroin. The former has accounted for about 10% of cases, while the latter has led to almost 80%; the remaining 10% were unclassified. The problems of AIDS-infected prostitutes are, in part, the fault of the growing tourist industry. The government has aroused public awareness and implemented preventive measures such as provision of condoms and blood tests for HIV-positive drug addicts, but there is an additional problem of social isolation. Moreover, there are few facilities for providing counselling and few places for known HIV-positive patients to live. They face very difficult lives in the community.

Mental health services

Mental health care in Thailand developed about a century ago. Mental health services are provided by psychiatric hospitals, mental health institutes and mobile community units distributed all over the country. Psychiatric institutions, psychiatric hospitals and centres, and psychiatric departments in general hospitals are under the Ministry of Public Health. There are also military and police hospitals, and university hospitals. Some private hospitals and clinics also accept psychiatric patients.

The first mental hospital was established in Bangkok in 1889. Later, the service was extended to the community through the establishment of mobile psychiatric units and psychiatric departments in some general hospitals. However, only a small minority of the population had access to these services, especially in rural areas. The co-ordination with other social services was far from adequate. Thus, the integration of mental health into the existing general health care system was promoted (Laksanavicharn, 1988*a*,*b*). Table 2.5 shows the distribution of hospitals and centres providing psychiatric services.

Table 2.6 shows the provision of psychiatric beds around the country. The bed occupancy rate is approximately 87.5% (Division of Mental Health, 1987).

The average length of stay reported from the Division of Mental Health is 68 days. The biggest mental hospital in Bangkok has reported an average of 82 days. The average length of stay is longer in the mental handicap

TABLE 2.5

Number of hospitals/centres providing psychiatric services divided by administration and region (1988)

Administration	Number
Department of medical services	
Division of mental health	
Bangkok (1 forensic psychiatric hospital, 1 mental handicap hospital, 1 mental health centre, 1 (biggest) mental hospital)	4
Central Region (excluding Bangkok) (1 hospital for autistic children, 1 community health centre, 1 psychiatric hospital)	3
Northern Region (1 neuropsychiatric hospital, 1 psychiatric hospital)	2
Southern Region (1 neuropsychiatric hospital, 1 psychiatric hospital)	2
North-eastern Region (3 psychiatric hospitals)	3
General hospitals	
Bangkok (1 hospital for children, 1 hospital for monks, 1 neuropsychiatric hospital, 1 general hospital)	4
Office of the Permanent Secretary of Public Health	
Central Region (excluding Bangkok)	19
Northern Region	6
Southern Region	7
North-eastern Region	7
(all are general hospitals)	
Ministry of Defence	
Medical Department of Army	
Bangkok (1 university hospital)	1
Central Region (excluding Bangkok) (2 hospitals for addiction)	2
Medical Department of Royal Air Force	
Bangkok (1 general hospital)	1
Ministry of Interior	
Thai National Police Department	
Bangkok (1 general hospital)	1
Bangkok Metropolis	
Bangkok (2 general hospitals, 5 mental health clinics)	7
Office of University Affairs	
Bangkok	3
Northern Region	1
Southern Region	1
North-eastern	1
(all are university hospitals)	

TABLE 2.6

Psychiatric bed provision in Thailand

Area	Population per bed	No. of beds per 10 000 population
Overall country	6879	1.45
Bangkok	2994	3.34
Other provinces	8093	1.24

hospital in Bangkok, which has reported an average of 2342 days. There are also places for long-stay patients in large mental hospitals.

The psychiatrist/population ratio is 1:393 235, being lowest in the northeastern region (1:699 455), and highest in Bangkok (1:121 947). The total number of psychiatrists in 1987 was 169 and the number of beds per psychiatrist was 62. The total number of nurses in mental health was 633 and the ratio of beds to nurses was 12:1.

Community outreach, community mental health centres, primary care centres

It is well known that the rural population has experienced little benefit from mental health services because of the poor distribution of health services in general, and mental health services in particular. Some general doctors deal with mental health problems where there is extreme scarcity of mental health workers.

Since resources in mental health services are limited, the Department of Medical Services has integrated mental health into the existing primary health care system as one of its ten essential elements. Activities in mental health include promotion, treatment, prevention, and rehabilitation. Pamphlets and posters providing mental health education are distributed. There are also rehabilitation centres established in different parts of the country to serve chronic patients and to develop technology in rehabilitation according to local culture and the needs of the population (Laksanavicharn, 1985).

Intersectoral participation

As yet, there is no formal participation with non-medical sectors. The judiciary may call on psychiatric experts and there is a forensic psychiatric hospital in Bangkok. Police throughout the country bring patients to care in emergencies. Efforts have been made to promote mental health education in schools and universities, some of which have psychiatrists and psychologists acting as counsellors.

Manpower and training

The number of psychiatrists and nurses has already been mentioned. There are about 60 psychologists employed in the Division of Mental Health. The number of mental health workers is very small. Of the total number of qualified practising psychiatrists throughout the country, the majority work in psychiatric institutions, university hospitals and departments of psychiatry in provincial general hospitals. Approximately 55% work in Bangkok while 45% are scattered in the provinces.

In 1988–89 the Thai Medical Council approved 28 posts for first-year residents in a three-year psychiatric residency training programme in seven institutions, leading to the certification of the Thai Board of Psychiatry.

Undergraduates are taught behavioural sciences in the first year at medical school and psychiatry during the second year. In addition, students have one term of lectures in clinical psychiatry in the third year and a one-month psychiatric clerkship in the fifth year.

There is a special training for nurses to qualify as psychiatric nurses. Most psychologists have had previous experience as teachers – training to become a teacher includes psychology.

From time to time, short courses and training are organised by universities and the Ministry of Public Health, for doctors, nurses and even mental health workers.

Epidemiological data

Most of the research is carried out in the universities and the Ministry of Public Health. The big hospitals, including those belonging to the medical schools, are overwhelmed with patients as there is neither a catchment area nor a systematic referral system. This situation restricts research. Epidemiological data are limited as there is neither enough trained staff nor a good data-collecting system.

During 1983–86 an increasing number of mentally ill patients attended government hospitals, but in 1987 the number decreased (Table 2.7).

TABLE 2.7
Number of psychiatric patients attending hospital

	1983	1984	1985	1986	1987
Whole kingdom	615 203	663 230	673 682	688 910	678 559

In 1986 the rate of attendance by people with mental illness at out-patient departments throughout Thailand was 21.0 per 1000 population. Mental illness has become one of the commonest reasons for attendance during the last five years. During 1983–1987 the suicide rate was more or less stable. In 1987 it was 5.8 per 100 000 population compared with 6.6 per 100 000 population in 1983 (Bussaratid & Ruangtrakool, 1983). The rate was consistently higher in men than women. In 1987 the North had the highest suicide rate and the North-eastern region the lowest rate.

The number of drug-dependent patients voluntarily attending treatment and rehabilitation centres is increasing. In 1983 the number was 60 323 (including 13 891 new cases). Over 95% of patients are men. Among new cases in 1989, there was an increase in the number of volatile substance users but a decrease in opium addicts. Most of the opiate addicts were found in Bangkok and large cities while very few were found in the Northern Region where the well known Golden Triangle is situated (Table 2.8).

TABLE 2.8
Number of narcotic addicts entering hospitals for treatment, classified by domicile (1989)

Region	Number (percentage of total)
Northern	7612 (12.62)
North-eastern	1966 (3.26)
Central	14 942 (24.77)
Southern	6165 (10.22)
Bangkok Metropolis	28 503 (47.25)
Foreigners and unidentifiable	1134 (1.88)
Total	60 323
Number of Narcotic Addicts Arrested	
1987	45 694
1986	39 234

Policies and programmes

The government has adopted the policy of providing nationwide accessibility to health services in order to achieve the goal of "Health for All by the Year 2000". In the fifth Five-Year National Health Plan (1982–1986), ideas of community mental health, deinstitutionalisation and the integration of mental health services into general health services were introduced. However, because of the resistance of conservative elements, such integration has never taken place.

Influenced by the Community Mental Health Centre Act of 1963 in the United States, Thailand introduced the so-called "open-door policy". Mobile psychiatric teams were first established in psychiatric hospitals, extending the service from hospitals to the community (Laksanavicharn, 1988*a,b*).

However, the lack of catchment areas, poor continuity of care and the overall insufficiency of services have presented difficulties. Therefore, since 1977–87 when interest in community care was greatest, there has been a return to the idea of institutionally based care using sophisticated technology.

Mental health legislation

There is no Mental Health Act in Thailand. Admissions and management are arranged informally between the psychiatrists, doctors, multidisciplinary teams and relatives.

Future problems and solutions

What are the problems?

As in other developing countries, there is a financial shortage and a lack of adequate local data on which to plan services.

The use of Western approaches and therapies is not entirely suitable to or acceptable in Thai culture (Mikulas, 1983). Furthermore, the mental health services are divided between different departments and divisions in the Ministry of Public Health.

Priorities

In 1984, the World Health Organization identified four main mental health priorities: emergencies, chronic major illness, problems associated with general medical care, and specific high-risk groups (such as alcohol and drug abusers) (Gelder *et al* 1989). Available resources should be concentrated on these areas. The reasonably successful Thai model managing the rehabilitation of the addictions should be used as an example of the management of chronic major psychiatric disorders. The management of psychiatric emergencies can be effectively improved by education and training of non-medical personnel to deal with them through simple measures supplemented by access to psychiatric expertise.

Psychiatry for all by the year 2000

The essential way of providing psychiatry for all by the year 2000 is for psychiatry to become an important specialty in medicine. It is also important to promote psychiatry and psychiatric approaches in non-medical areas of society such as education, the media, religion, occupations and the social sector.

Primary health care

To incorporate mental health into primary health care, mental health professionals should become members of a health team or work in the general health care system as a consultant, an educator or a collaborator. This approach will allow consultations with general health professionals to decrease physical illness associated with psychiatric morbidity.

There is also hope that, in the near future, crisis intervention units will be established in the community with well trained district health workers. Even at the village level, volunteers can help in screening and providing regular support, under supervision from mental health workers.

Evaluation of services

Two approaches should be adopted in the evaluation of services. One is to study the use of services within defined populations. The other is to carry out trials of different kinds of treatment.

Culture and mental health

Confounding cultural influences can disrupt mental health care. In the Thai culture, it is more acceptable for someone with psychological problems to talk to monks rather than medical professionals. There is also a belief in karma – that one's current life situation is to some extent dependent on one's actions in the past life. Therefore, an individual passively accepts some aspects of his or her life situation. This in turn leads to less tendency to consult services.

Personnel training – who, where and how many?

Personnel training is one of the most important developments in providing services. The training should include every level of manpower.

In the medical profession, training in mental health can be categorised into three levels:

(a) Physicians, nurses and health officers located in the province or district
(b) Health workers at middle level such as junior health workers, midwives, etc.
(c) Community health workers such as VHCs and VHVs.

The role of international agencies and developed countries

The government should work hand in hand with the responsible agencies both inside and outside the country. Funding from abroad should be in the form of funds for internal projects on prevention, treatment and rehabilitation, research, and training.

References

BUSSARATID, S. & RUANGTRAKOOL, S. (1983) Thailand. In *Suicide in Asia and the Near-east* (ed. L. A. Headley). Berkeley: University of California Press.

DIVISION OF HEALTH STATISTICS (1985) *Public Health Statistics*. Bangkok: Ministry of Public Health.

GELDER, M., GATH, D. & MAYOU, R. (1989) *Oxford Textbook of Psychiatry* (2nd edn). Oxford: Oxford University Press.

LAKSANAVICHARN, U. (1985) Mental health services in Thailand during the fifth five-year national health plan (1982–1986). *Journal of the Psychiatric Association of Thailand*, **30**, 1–4.

—— (1988a) Some aspects of the mental health care programme in Thailand. *Bulletin of the Department of Medical Services*, **13**, 69–70.

—— (1988b) Psychiatric training for serving the community. *Journal of the Psychiatric Association of Thailand*, **33**, 239–241.

MIKULAS, W. (1983) Thailand and behaviour modification. *Journal of Behavioural Therapy and Experimental Psychiatry*, **14**, 93–97.

OFFICE OF THE NATIONAL ECONOMIC AND SOCIAL DEVELOPMENT BOARD (1987) *Social Indicators in 10 years and Social Indicators*. Bangkok: ONESDB.

WORLD HEALTH ORGANIZATION (1978) *Mental Disorders: Glossary and Guide to their Classification in Accordance with the Ninth Revision of the International Classification of Diseases (ICD–9)*. Geneva: WHO.

3 Korea: looking for change

JUNG IM SHIM

Land, people and culture

Korea, so-called 'Land of Morning Calm', is a peninsula located in the furthest part of the Far East. Its northern extremity is adjacent to the Sino-Soviet border, i.e. Manchuria and Siberia. To the west, Korea faces China across the Yellow Sea, and to the south lies the Pacific Ocean, while to the east, the Sea of Japan separates Korea from the Japanese archipelago. Most of the country (70%) is mountainous, particularly the north and the east coast. The major agricultural resources, including rice, are found in the southeast plain. The total area of North and South Korea is about 85 000 square miles – slightly smaller than Great Britain. There are four distinct seasons; each July the monsoon brings heavy rains and causes flooding. Korean is a member of the Altaic family of languages, which includes Tungusic, Turkish and Mongolian. When earlier waves of migrants entered Korea around the third millennium BC they drove the natives, the Paleosians, north to Sakhalin, Kamchatka and the Arctic region. A few were assimilated with the new settlers. For hundreds of years Koreans used Chinese characters for writing but King Sejong (1399–1450), with the aid of court scholars, invented a useful phonetic system of writing for transcribing the Korean language and named it *'Hangul'*.

South Korea has a large population for a small territory; it totals 42 380 000 people, of whom a quarter live in Seoul. The crude birth rate was 19.1 per 10 000 persons in 1987. Article 81 of the Law of Education, which was promulgated in 1949 and amended in 1951, provides for the establishment of seven types of school or college so that all citizens receive equal opportunities for education regardless of their religion, sex, or socio-economic status. Illiteracy appears to be unusual. The economic development of Korea has been remarkable during the past two decades, especially following the Korean War. Urban–rural differences are apparent, and better sanitation, housing and facilities can be found in large towns but cities such as Seoul suffer from poor housing.

History

The Three Kingdoms period

The Tangun was believed to have founded the ancient Chosun Kingdom in 2333 BC. In the course of time, small tribal states developed into the Three Kingdoms: Kogurryo, Paekche and Silla. Kogurryo, which occupied the northern part of the peninsula, was the first to receive Buddhism and Confucianism from China. Buddhism was officially recognised as the national religion of Kogurryo in AD 372. Paekche, for geopolitical reasons, is thought to have exerted a powerful influence on the development of Japanese culture during the 4th and 5th centuries. Competition between the three kingdoms ended with the unified Korean Kingdom of Silla in AD 676, for which credit is due to Wang Kon, the founder of a dynasty that came to be known as the Koryo Dynasty. The name *Korea* itself is derived from *Koryo*.

The dynasties of Koryo and Yi

The Koryo enjoyed relative peace until it was invaded by the Mongols in AD 1231, and was famous for its art, especially ceramics. In 1368, Yi-Song Gae, one of the leading generals, established the Yi Dynasty by a *coup d'état*. This lasted for over 500 years until Korea was annexed by Japan in 1910.

The Japanese colonial rule

Western powers penetrated Korea during the latter part of the 19th century, eyeing Korea's resources and its rich harvest of rice. While the Korean king at that time strenuously opposed foreign influences, Korea was compelled to sign treaties of friendship and commerce, first with Japan in 1876, then the United States in 1882, Britain and Germany in 1883, Italy and Russia in 1884, and France in 1886.

Japan established firm control over the country, having won wars against China and Russia that had been fought on Korean soil in 1894–95 and 1904 respectively. By 1910, Japan had abandoned the pretence that Korea was a protectorate, and declared it to be a colony in order to legitimise the total exploitation of the country. Throughout the period of Japanese rule, 1910–45, the Korean people demonstrated several times against its ruthlessness.

After liberation

In 1945, at the end of World War II, arrangements were made for the Japanese to surrender to the Soviet Union in the northern part of Korea and to the United States in the South. When North Korea invaded the South on 25 June 1950, 16 nations entered the Korean War under the flag of the UN to help the defence of South Korea. The country was devastated. In the ceasefire of 1953, the peninsula was divided into the north and the south by a demilitarised zone which followed the 38th parallel.

Government and political situation

A modern political system was introduced at the end of World War II in the Republic of Korea. The system had previously centred on an absolute monarchy in which a king had the ultimate decision-making power in administrative and judicial affairs. However, from 1945–48 the Republic of Korea became independent.

Korea now has a presidential system of government with a unicameral legislature called the National Assembly. The president is the apex of government, the head of state, the chief executive and the leader of the ruling party. He is elected by direct vote for a single five-year term.

Government is highly centralised; the provincial and municipal governments are not yet fully independent from the national government. Governors and mayors are appointed by the President.

Since the killing of former dictator Park, and of his successor Chun for his part in the 1982 "Kwang Ju massacre", Korean politics has been unsettled.

Health services in the Republic of Korea

Structure and organisation

Government level

The Ministry of Health and Social Affairs (MHSA) is a government body which consists of one Assistant Minister for Planning and Management, seven Bureaux, 28 departments and seven officers. Its functional divisions are public health, sanitation, medical affairs, medical insurance, national pension, pharmaceutical affairs and home welfare. The following institutions are regulated by the MHSA: three National Mental Hospitals, one National Medical Centre, three National Hospitals for Tuberculosis, and 13 Quarantine Centres. The Red Cross is also an associated organisation. The annual budget is relatively small compared to that of the Ministry of Military Defence, and is audited by the Economic Planning Board.

Provincial level in city and country

Every city and province has a Bureau for Health and Social Affairs, each with five departments similar to those of the MHSA. This dual administration system hinders the efficiency of the health service.

The director of a health centre is nominated by the mayor or governor and is unlikely to be a doctor, as not many doctors want to work in primary health care with its poorly paid and poorly run system of management. A more even distribution of medical manpower is one of the priorities for the future of health care delivery in Korea. The director of a health centre is important in decision-making, arranging for patients to be referred to the upper levels of health care (Cho, 1982).

District level in villages

Each village has one sub-health centre for primary health care and referrals. Nurse-practitioners are assigned to work in primary care following two years of special training. This was originally intended to compensate for the shortage of doctors at 'grass-roots' level, but it has yet to make a major impression.

Medical facilities

There are 519 hospitals in Korea. Only 55 belong to the public sector, while the rest are in the private sector. Ambulatory clinics are now increasing their facilities relative to hospitals. The nurses and medical professions are also rapidly increasing in number. Almost 40% of doctors practise in Seoul, although health authorities have tried to increase the numbers outside the capital. This overcentralisation is one of the serious obstacles in achieving the goal of 'Health for All'. There are relatively few public health workers, and salaries are lower than in the private sector.

The goals of accessibility and affordability have not yet been universally achieved. Access to care is still limited. Civil servants and their families, teachers, students and soldiers can be provided for by health services through the medical insurance card. But farmers, fishermen and labourers who do not belong to a company or any government organisations are often not eligible to use the card.

Mental health services

There are three mental hospitals under the MHSA in Korea with a total of 1900 beds. In addition, all general hospitals have psychiatric departments. However, there is no separate administration for mental health. By law, mental health services must be provided in every health centre, although this is not fully enforced.

Personnel

There are 300 psychiatrists but no specially trained psychiatric nurses. Psychologists have two major roles in practice: clinical psychology and psychoanalysis. In villages, health workers, in addition to their roles in health education and prevention, also detect the mentally ill by home visits.

Psychiatric trainees join hospitals registered with the Korean Hospitals Association, which regulates the number of trainees and supervises their training programmes. Trainees spend three years gaining the required professional experience.

Approaches to mental health

Korean psychiatry was originally influenced by Japanese disciples of Kraepelin during the 36 years of colonial rule, and after the Korean war, dynamic psychiatry was introduced by the Americans. Since 1958, the training programme has been the same as in the United States: internship and residency. In the 1960s, Korean psychiatrists were interested in cultural and social psychiatry and studied the prevalence of mental illness (Yu, 1962). The concepts of mental illness and illness behaviour were debated keenly (Kim, 1974; Choi, 1974; Rhi, 1986).

By the 1980s, the Neuropsychiatry Association was prominent. One of its concerns was the facilities for chronic patients and the use of locked wards. Drafts of a mental health act were revised and submitted to the government. However, anti-government politicians saw a possible political abuse of restraining legislations and the parliamentary General Assembly finally dismissed the proposal.

There are increasing numbers of government officials who recognise mental health problems to be important and to require financial support, and community-based treatment and rehabilitation. Yet, discrepancies between government proposals and those of mental health professionals still exist.

The impact of culture on mental health services and mental illness

The tradition of looking after the disabled is deeply rooted in Korean culture. Medicine was administered by the government from the Three Kingdom period (Kim, 1966). After World War II, Western culture poured into Korea. Rapid industrialisation led to cohesiveness of the family and neglect of traditional mores, and spiritual values. Since then, overcentralised policy and bureaucracy have hindered the development of mental health services.

Disorders similar to those in the West are found. According to Lee's findings (Lee, 1990) on the lifetime prevalence of DSM–III disorders (American Psychiatric Association, 1980) in Seoul, there is a high prevalence of alcohol abuse and alcohol dependence. The prevalence of schizophrenia and schizophreniform disorders is low, 0.34%; for affective disorders the figure is 5.52%. Anxiety and somatoform disorders are less common than in the United States while the prevalence of panic disorders and obsessive–compulsive disorders is similar. Anorexia nervosa is uncommon, only one case being found among a study of 3134 community subjects.

A disorder called *"Hwat-Byung"* is recognised, although not described in the English language literature. It may be thought of as a Korean "culture-bound syndrome" or a variant of major depression (Lin, 1983). This Korean folk illness is ordinarily understood by patients and families to be a physical affliction despite the fact that its manifestations include both physiological and psychological symptoms. In addition, the patient often recognises interpersonal conflicts and anger as precipitating factors. An understanding of the cultural context is indispensable in the diagnosis of *Hwat-Byung*. Despite the presence of psychological and behavioural symptoms such as insomnia, excessive tiredness, acute panic, morbid fear of impending death, and dysphoric mood, patients typically dwell more on their physical complaints, which include indigestion, anorexia, dyspnoea, palpitation, generalised pains and aches, and the feeling that there is a mass in the epigastrium. The somatic preoccupations are resistant to medical reassurance. Somatisation appears to be a common way for the distress of patients with psychiatric problems to be communicated.

The future of Korean mental health services

Mental health policy

It is most important that the government recognises that the needs of the chronically mentally ill are an important issue. Day centres, halfway houses and sheltered workshops are badly needed. Better training of all health workers in mental health is required.

Attitude of the general population

Korean people have varying attitudes to mental health depending on their sociocultural background, level of education, religion and personal experience. The stigma of mental illness has not disappeared, either for the general public or for government officials. Education of all social groups should be directed at increasing knowledge of illness, treatment and prevention (Shim, 1982).

Academic needs

Korean mental health services could be greatly improved by implementation of the following proposals:

(a) Evaluation of and research into the effectiveness of mental health in practice

(b) Establishment of a department of mental health in the MHSA and National Institute of Mental Health

(c) An overseas training scheme for mental health workers: an exchange programme to obtain expertise in countries with developed systems.

References

AHN, D. H. (1986) Community leader's attitude to mental illness. *Seoul Journal of Psychiatry*, **11**, 281–297.

AMERICAN PSYCHIATRIC ASSOCIATION (1980) *Diagnostic and Statistical Manual of Mental Disorders* (DSM–III) (3rd edn). Washington, DC: APA.

CHO, D. Y. (1982) Community supporting system for the mentally ill. *Bulletin of the Royal College of Psychiatrists*, **6**, 170–176.

CHOI, S. H. (1974) The concept of mental health. *Journal of Korean Medical Association*, **17**, 147–152.

KIM, D. J. (1966) *The History of Medicine in Korea*. Tamkudang, Seoul: Tam Kudang.

KIM, E. Y. *et al* (1974) A proposal for the medical delivery system for the mentally ill in Korea. *Korean Mental Health*, **4**, 244–266.

LEE, C. K. *et al* (1990) Psychiatric epidemiology in Korea. *Journal of Nervous and Mental Disease*, **178**, 242–246.

LIN, K. M. (1983) Hwa-Byung: a Korean culture-bound syndrome? *American Journal of Psychiatry*, **140**, 105–107.

RHI, B. Y. *et al* (1985) A preliminary study about health-seeking behaviour of the mentally ill. *Journal of Korean Neuro-Psychiatry*, **28**, 307–324.

SHIM, J. I. (1982) The psychosocial approach to the mentally ill in Korea. In *Textbook of Health Management* (ed. S. C. Oh), pp. 257–269. Park Young Co.

SHIM, J. I. (1989) The introduction of the Mental Health Act in England and Wales. *Journal of Law and Psychiatry*, **2**, 281–303.

YU, S. J. (1962) Mental disorders in Korean rural communities. *Journal of Korean Neuro-psychiatry*, **1**, 9–27.

II. Europe

4 Italy: the post-1978 reform era – difficulties, dilemmas and future directions

CHIARA SAMELE and CARLO BOLOGNA

Over the past decade, psychiatric care in Italy has been the subject of much debate, following the inception of what is regarded as a revolutionary piece of mental health legislation in 1978 (Mosher, 1982). An abundance of reports can be found in the literature (De Girolamo, 1989), reflecting the interest generated by Italy's reform.

Italy itself consists of 20 regions. Fig. 4.1 shows the country according to region and major cities. The total population in 1989 reached 57 436 000. Italy has the lowest birth rate in Europe, 9.6% in 1989 compared with the EC average of 11.8%. The rate is lower in the north than in the south. The southern birth rate is estimated to grow as a proportion of Italy's total birth rate from 36% at present to more than 40% in 2010. Projections for the same year predict a decrease in population of one million. Table 4.1 shows the percentage age distribution for 1988.

The death rate per 1000 population in 1987 was 9.3. The major causes of death per 100 000 population in 1986 were diseases of the circulatory system 421.4; malignant neoplasms (cancers) 236.7; diseases of the respiratory system 66.9 and digestive system 52.4.

The distribution of the population in the first 25 years of Italy's post-war industrial and economic boom meant mass migration from the south to find work both in northern cities and other industrial countries. Migration on a grand scale has generally stopped. The country is now beginning to experience immigration which is due to lax visa controls making entry relatively easy compared to other European Community (EC) countries. Italy now has about 1–1.5 million immigrants, mainly from Northern Africa.

Italy is the fifth biggest economy in the world. Despite the wealth it enjoys, it is also markedly poor. The contrast is evident when comparing certain regions of the north such as Lombardy and Piedmont to those of the south like Campania, Calabria and Sicily. In economic terms, the south is much worse off. For example, in 1988 unemployment for northerners was 7.7% compared to 21% in the south. Overall, Italy has a higher rate of unemployment (currently 10.8%) than any other EC economy apart from

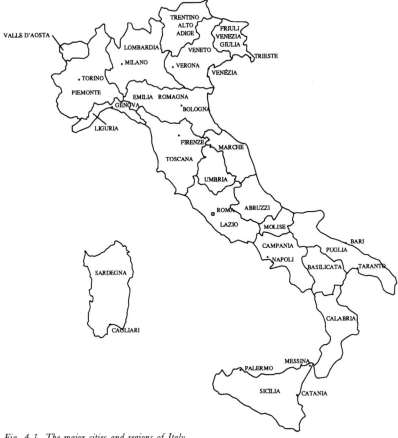

Fig. 4.1. The major cities and regions of Italy

TABLE 4.1
Age distribution (%) of the Italian population in 1988

	Age: years					
	under 15	15–29	30–44	45–59	60–74	75 +
Percentage of population	17.8	24.1	20.1	18.6	13.5	5.9

Spain. The workforce at present is 25 million. Output per head in the south is 56% of that in the north. Although the south is poorer, consumption was 87% of the national average in 1987. This was made possible by vast government transfer payments, highlighting the dependency of the south on the rest of the country. It is a dependency that has grown during the 1980s, exacerbating the budget deficit, and further heightened by the estimate that 45% of Italy's total value added tax goes uncollected. ISTAT (1987) officially put the size of the 'economia sommersa' (submerged economy) at 18% of gross domestic product (GDP). Public sector borrowing (PSB) in 1985 was nearly 15% of GDP.

Italy's political background has been described as 'volatile stability' (Grimond, 1990). When the prime minister, Giulio Andreotti, came to power in July 1989, his was the 50th government since 1945. The most prominent political party is the Democrazia Cristiana (Christian Democrat). The Communist Party has been a feature of post-war coalition governments and, following a restructuring, is likely to adopt a more social democratic approach. In the 1980s the Socialist Party, headed by Bettino Craxi, became the main contender for the Communist vote.

Development of Italy's national health service

The legislative enactment of a national health service in Italy in 1978 (Servizio Sanitario Nazionale, SSN) not only introduced a more comprehensive system of health care, but was later to incorporate the new system of mental health care, despite coming from a separate law.

Health care before the 1978 reform was insurance based, and approximately 200 sickness funds provided cover for about 90% of the population. The remaining 10% not covered by these schemes, for reasons of non-eligibility (e.g. the chronically mentally ill), were able to apply for means-tested social assistance administered by provincial authorities.

The campaign for a comprehensive system of health care was led by the trade union movement and the political Left. Gross inequalities in the distribution of health services around the country existed, which the government recognised as needing decisive action. The most fundamental concern of central ministries, however, was containing health expenditure, although the amount of GDP earmarked for health care was approximately 5%, which represented one of the lowest within EC countries (Ramon, 1985).

The regions are designated to establish, maintain and administer services, and secure the effective distribution of central government's financial expenditure among the health service sectors. The law led to the formation of Local Health Units (Unitá Sanitaria Locale, USL) to organise health services. USLs are responsible for the functioning of socio-health services and liaise with associated welfare services within the confines of local government communes.

A population covered by a USL is generally between 40 000 and 200 000 people. Each USL is divided into districts with a population of around 10 000, providing basic health services, including primary care, family advice centres, pharmacies and some domiciliary services. Specialised health services are provided for the USL as a whole. Detailed arrangements often vary from one health district to another. A USL with an effective provision of services (often found in a northern city) is divided into three main sections: health, social services and administration. The number of health care staff is set, as a maximum for each district of 10 000 people, at: six doctors, four social workers, four psychologists and 12 nurses (Robb, 1986).

Money for the health service comes from the National Health Fund (Fondo Sanitario Nazionale) and forms part of the annual state budget. The fund is divided into two parts, one concerning capital works, the other operating costs. Much of the fund derives its income from insurance contributions paid by employers and employees, and various health-related organisations. In addition, the service is supported by general taxation. However, during the initial stages of implementation, Italy was undergoing a deep economic recession where the costs for health care were increasingly being drawn from general taxation. Soon patients themselves became more accountable for treatment costs as personal contributions were extended. Cuts in health expenditure totalled 20% in 1982 (Mangen, 1989).

Implementation of health services has been slow in some regions and even where areas have been successful it is evident that funds still pay the high cost of in-patient care while preventive and community services suffer. The health service is dependent upon doctors being willing to work free of charge to gain experience, in view of the high unemployment rate among doctors, and the fierce competition for medical posts (Mangen, 1989).

Health services are becoming progressively dispersed among public, voluntary and private agencies, each seeking to guard its own ground. This adds to the increasing problems of co-ordination which can be traced to the health and social policies over the past 15 years (Donati, 1985). In a large city, several USLs may exist, each with its own budget and following its own policies, although keeping in line with regional plans. Inevitably, this makes the operation and monitoring of health services somewhat convoluted, especially as communities have no control over them.

In the short term, the prospects for improving the National Health service appear bleak, given that an increasing amount of the health budget goes towards meeting the demand for health care rather than improving the service's functioning. Assessments of the effectiveness of the health service during its first decade of application have been unfavourable, and one report estimates that more than half of the population seeks private health care (Martino, 1986).

Plans for modifying the health service again are attempts to curb the ascending costs and have included the idea of introducing a three-tier system whereby higher income groups would pay for the entire cost of their treatment. Such income groups would simply resort to private treatment.

The problems of the National Health service, despite the proposals for change, still require definite solutions and whatever these are, they will have direct consequences for the psychiatric services.

Mental health legislation before 1978
and the context for change

Italy's first piece of psychiatric legislation, passed in 1904, requested that each province provide a mental asylum. This law had two contradictory aims. The first was a custodial–repressive one to regulate, by means of a set of public safety rules, the commitment of the mentally deranged whose behaviour disturbed the peace, or who could be a danger to themselves or others. The second was a humanitarian objective to rectify and prevent the abuse of patients in asylums and replace these with more suitable environments to facilitate recovery.

The humanitarian/welfare purpose became more explicit in the 1909 Regulations, enforced as an adjunct to the 1904 law. These regulations sought to limit the excess numbers of patients admitted to institutions, to promote a more sanitary environment and abolish (or use only in exceptional cases) mechanical restraints.

Following the presentation of several bills to Parliament from 1951 and pressure by the Association of Italian Psychiatric Hospital Doctors, Italy's second mental health legislation was enacted in 1968. This introduced for the first time the concept of voluntary admissions for purposes of diagnosis and treatment. There was also provision to change the admission status of a patient from a compulsory to a voluntary basis.

The outcome of the war and the years immediately following had set in motion a fundamental questioning of all that had previously been accepted, including the role of the Catholic Church and the State in society.

This era of reform was volatile owing to pressures brought to bear by a variety of groups, such as the women's, the trade union and the students' movements, emerging in the early 1970s. The formation of Psichiatria Democratica (Democratic Psychiatry, PD) in 1973 began a movement which struggled against the marginalisation of the mentally ill. Political parties during this time, particularly those of the Left, joined in consolidating the pressure for social reforms through Parliamentary legislation, leading to laws for divorce, abortion, reform in mental health and the formation of a national health service.

Underlying philosophy for reforming mental health care

The incentive for transforming Italy's mental health system came with the founding of Psichiatria Democratica by Franco Basaglia and his wife Franca Ongaro-Basaglia, who initiated serious opposition to institutional practices in mental health care. The formation of this formal organisation aimed to defray many of the models and achievements in experiments of de-institutionalisation initiated in 1961 in Gorzia by Basaglia and his co-workers (Schepher-Hughes & Lovell, 1986). The movement's original pledges consisted of the following:

(a) To continue to fight prejudice against psychiatric patients both in the workplace and elsewhere
(b) To struggle against the asylum as the most obvious and violent paradigm of exclusion
(c) To avoid reproducing institutional mechanisms for exclusion in the community
(d) To make clear the link between health and mental health care, especially through the reform of the Italian health care system (Schepher-Hughes & Lovell, 1986, p.167).

Many of PD's objectives and underlying ideology were detailed in a book edited by Basaglia in 1967 entitled *L'Istituzione Negata* ("The Institution Denied"). Here, the basic philosophy was moving the pivot of the 'psychiatric response' from the hospital to the community (territorio[1]) in the belief that the hospital as the 'total' answer becomes a significant cause of chronicity and of social exclusion and that only a flexible and diversified range of non-hospital responses can assume a therapeutic and rehabilitative role. What is thus described is a wide 'circle' of comprehensive intervention taking place in various settings outside the hospital. The basic character of such comprehensive intervention is that of 'therapeutic continuity', i.e. the same team of professionals provides each different stage of care.

Enacting the 1978 mental health reform

The 1978 Mental Health Reform Act was drafted and passed in haste during a coalition government. The Radical Party (a small but influential party of the Left) sponsored PD's campaign in Parliament with the use of a national referendum that required the collection of 500 000 signatures, which according to the Italian constitution would uproot the 1904 mental health legislation, leaving the status of mental hospitals in disarray. Thus efforts by both PD and the Radical Party managed to amass enough signatures to cause the government political embarrassment, as experienced previously with divorce and abortion, which it was at pains to avoid. The Mental Health Act was passed in May 1978, much of it a compromise of opinions. Its enactment was not only rapid but also performed without prior investigation or evaluation. The principal features of Law 180 include the following:

(a) A gradual phasing out of public mental hospitals by prohibiting any further admissions to them. A deadline set for December 1980 (31 December 1981 in some areas) continued to allow ex-mental hospital patients to be readmitted on a voluntary basis, after which admission became unlawful.

---

1. It should be noted that the difference between *community* and *territory* refers to the Italian concept of home/natural environment care of the patient and not in terms of community facilities such as hostels, recreational centres, local authority residential homes, etc.

The construction of mental hospitals was outlawed and existing psychiatric hospitals were to take discharged patients.

Staff for new services were to be drawn from personnel of mental hospitals (this acted as a redeployment of staff).

The status of in-patients was to be reassessed to determine whether continued commitment was deemed necessary and to specify the probable duration of treatment.

(b) In general, treatment would ordinarily take place outside the hospital in community-based facilities responsible for a pre-defined geographical area. These facilities would be organised to safeguard collaboration between general and mental hospitals in order to provide both preventive and rehabilitative psychiatric interventions.

(c) Hospital admission, whether on a voluntary or compulsory basis, was to be used as a last resort. General hospital psychiatric wards (Servizi Psichiatrici di Diagnosi e Cura, SPDC) were to be set up for all in-patient treatment. The number of beds available in each unit/ward was to be limited to 15 per 200 000 population and based in community mental health centres (Centro di Salute Mentale, CSM) and/or the SPDC.

(d) Compulsory admission to private hospitals was to be discontinued. Compulsory commitment to SPDCs for evaluation and treatment could occur if i) urgent intervention was essential, ii) treatment was refused, and iii) treatment in the community was not feasible. Two doctors' certificates were required (one of which had to be an independent evaluation).

The length of compulsory hospital admission was limited to seven days, subject to review at the second and seventh days. Applications for an extension had to be made to an independent judicial review. Appeals to court could be made by patients or relatives. The constitutional rights of involuntary patients had to be upheld.

This law does not apply to Italy's six forensic psychiatric hospitals, private hospitals, residential homes or nursing homes, and services primarily for substance abusers. The restructuring of mental health services aimed largely to desegregate the mentally ill, the mentally handicapped and the physically handicapped. The purpose of closing mental hospitals was to ensure that patients' lifestyles could be similar to those of other people. There were also attempts to shift away from the hegemony of medically trained staff to distribute power and responsibility equally among all professionals involved. Law 180 promoted the integration of psychiatry into the rest of medicine. The state and local authorities had to develop alternatives to the mental hospital.

The short conversion period from the enactment of Law 180 to the prohibition deadline for compulsory admissions to mental hospitals was purposely designed in order to prevent prolonged implementation.

Implementing Law 180

Full implementation of the reform required two preliminary conditions, as Basaglia (1967) outlined. The first was vigorous transformation inside the *manicomio* of its organisation and rapport with patients. These existing large mental hospitals can now be used for voluntary admissions, and although in some cases this can become long term, this is in fact an abuse of Law 180.

The second was a thorough programme aiming to move psychiatry beyond the walls of the *manicomio* and implement new 'agencies' in order to respond to needs in the community and 'weave' a network of functional links with health and social staff (i.e. GPs, social workers, home helps), families, local authorities, voluntary organisations, etc. (Tranchina, 1979).

The reform made a notable impact on the decline in numbers of both patients and beds in mental hospitals. Table 4.2 shows the reduction in the number of beds and patient figures from public mental hospitals and private psychiatric institutions between 1967 and 1984.

TABLE 4.2
Discharges from public mental hospitals and private psychiatric institutions[1]

Year	Public mental hospitals		Private psychiatric institutions	
	No. of beds	No. of patients[1]	No. of beds	No. of patients[1]
1967	91 594	86 063	23 037	20 116
1972	85 000	77 987	26 278	22 042
1977	70 070	58 445	24 177	19 663
1981	47 871	38 358	21 905	16 872
1984	38 928	30 672	18 345	15 025

(Source: ISTAT 1964–86)

1. Patients on census day, 31 December of previous year.

The rate of decrease in the number of beds in mental hospitals occurred fairly consistently between 1963 and 1968 and averaged 1390 beds per year. In the period between 1973 and 1978, before the reform, the rate was 3305. The post-reform years between 1979 and 1983 showed a 4140 per year reduction in beds (Tansella & Williams, 1987). Length of stay in state mental hospitals, however, showed an increase from 142 days to 236 days during 1977–1984. It could be argued that those patients who were suitable for discharge had left hospital before 1978, while the more severe cases, or those who would not benefit from discharge from hospital, remained. Admissions to state psychiatric hospitals in 1972 totalled 102 617 and by 1984 had decreased to 15 995 – said to be partly due to administrative artefacts (Mosher & Burti, 1989).

The number of patients in private institutions had also peaked in 1972, reaching a total of 22 042. Again this figure declined in the following years to 15 025 in 1984. Length of stay in private mental hospitals averaged 127 days in 1972 and decreased to an average of 87 days in 1984.

Types and distribution of psychiatric services in Italy

Table 4.3 lists the types and number of mental health services that exist.

TABLE 4.3
Types of psychiatric services existing in 1984

Types	Number
Public mental hospitals	89
Private mental hospitals	11
Private psychiatric institutions	87
University departments[1]	27
Forensic psychiatric hospitals	6
Residential Facilities[2]	248
Workers' Cooperatives	50
CSMs[3]	675
SPDCs	236

1. Approximately half of the university departments operate as SPDCs with 15 beds.
2. These facilities are alternatives to mental hospitals and do not include group homes. In 1984 these facilities had 2901 residents.
3. Day hospitals are often located within CSMs.
(Source: CENSIS, 1985; ISTAT, 1964–86; Mosher & Burti, 1989)

Referrals to psychiatric services can be through general practitioners (GPs) to a CSM, by relatives or the individuals themselves. In cases of emergency, referrals are via the general hospital to a SPDC.

Three models of Italian psychiatric care have been described by several authors (McCarthy, 1985; Misiti, 1985; Pirella, 1987) and can also be considered as stages of implementation. The first is typified by the persistence of mental hospitals or *manicomios*, reliance on SPDCs (which alone are not sufficient to meet the population's needs) and the predominance of private psychiatric facilities. Community services are few, or non-existent. Such services are found mainly in the south where service delivery is poor and inadequately developed. The second model is based on out-patient services with a small number of private facilities. Non-hospital residential and rehabilitation facilities are either underdeveloped or absent, with a continued reliance on hospital-orientated psychiatric care. This model can be recognised in northern and central regions and forms the major part of psychiatric care in Italy. The block in admissions to *manicomios* does apply, but those patients admitted before the reform are still accommodated within them.

The third model is essentially community-based services with almost no use of the mental hospital, which is either virtually empty or closed completely, and a limited use of SPDCs. The focal point of this model of

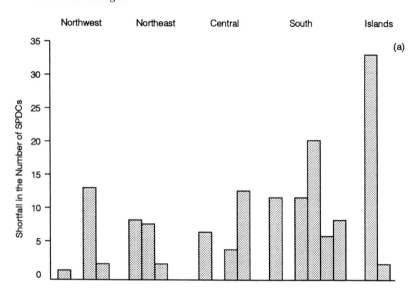

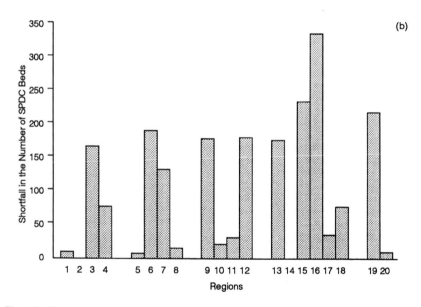

Fig. 4.2. The planned and operational (a) SPDCs and (b) SPDC beds by region in Italy. The regions are (1) Piemonte, (2) Valle d'Aosta, (3) Lombardia, (4) Liguria, (5) Trentino Alto Adige, (6) Veneto, (7) Friuli Venezia Giulia, (8) Emiglia Romagna, (9) Toscana, (10) Umbria, (11) Marche, (12) Lazio, (13) Abruzzo, (14) Molise, (15) Campania, (16) Puglia, (17) Basilicata, (18) Calabria, (19) Sicilia, (20) Sardegna (CENSIS, 1984, 1985)

care highlights services such as CSMs, sheltered flats, therapeutic communities, hostels, day centres, sheltered workshops and domiciliary visits. It is implemented in areas such as Trieste, South Verona, Perugia, Venice, Turin, Genoa and Portoguaro (Martini *et al*, 1985; Gallio & Giannichedda, 1982).

Let us evaluate the implementation of psychiatric services, and the spread of SPDCs and community services such as CSMs, following the reform.

SPDCs

Figure 4.2*a* shows the gap in the number of SPDCs both planned and operational. The shortfall in the number of SPDCs (wards) by region tends to predominate in southern areas such as Puglia and Sicilia.

Similarly, the shortfall in the number of SPDC beds, shown in Fig. 4.2*b*, becomes more marked in the same regions, including Campania.

In assessing compliance with the reform, Mosher & Burti (1989) show that, on average, each service has 13 beds, two fewer than the estimated figure of 15 specified in Law 180. They point out that in accordance with the generally accepted ratio of 1 bed per 1000 population, some 173 new units would have to be developed with approximately 2595 new beds.

An estimated 78 000 admissions take place each year in SPDCs. One-fifth of these admissions are compulsory. The average length of stay in SPDCs is approximately 12 days, with little difference between voluntary and compulsory admissions. Readmissions amount to one-third (34.1%) of the total admissions figure (Mosher & Burti, 1989; CENSIS, 1985 data).

Staff make-up and the distribution of personnel in SPDCs again show an uneven spread across the country, with a high proportion of medically orientated facilities and a general lack of formal training for staff in new services, with only one-third of regions offering courses. Those professionals who have transferred from mental hospitals to new services constitute 58.6% of all mental health professionals, those employed after the reform make up 23%, and the remaining 15% come from other services. Staff composition in SPDCs is 69.7% psychiatric nurses, 21.7% physicians, 3.8% social workers, and 4.0% psychologists.

Community psychiatric services in Italy

Centros di Salute Mentale (CSMs) are the cornerstone of psychiatric services in Italy, according to the ideals of Law 180. As of December 1984, 674 community psychiatric services have functioned in Italy, with a total number of 360 000 users that year, 33% of whom were first contacts. The number of these services, distributed by region, is shown in Fig. 4.3.

Essentially, they offer a 'walk-in' service, run on an informal basis so that people can attend without an appointment. Other responsibilities of the CSM include domiciliary visits by staff members, assessments, drug

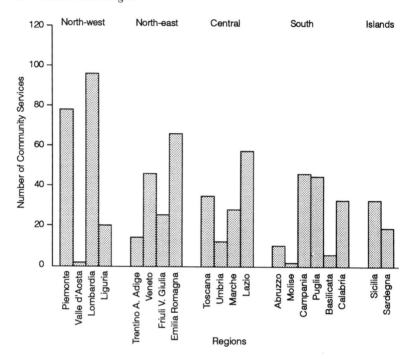

Fig. 4.3. Community psychiatric services in Italy by region (CENSIS, 1984, 1985)

prescriptions and psychotherapeutic meetings. Some centres have beds for overnight stay and most are open six days a week.

The unequal distribution of community services can be seen when considering the ratio of services to population. In the north the ratio is one service per 70 000 population. In central regions there is one service per 80 000 population, in the south one service per 100 000 population, and in Sicily, one per 149 000 population. Drastic discrepancies are found between Friuili Venezia Giulia (northeast), with one service per 47 000 population, and Molise (south) with one service per 333 000 population (CENSIS, 1985, cited in Mosher & Burti, 1989).

Of the existing community services, 37% were created before the 1978 reform; once Law 180 was introduced the trend increased until 1980 and subsequently slowed down. Some 132 community services are still lacking and approximately one-third of the population live in USLs without psychiatric services in the community (Mosher & Burti, 1989).

Only one-third of community services in Italy have all professionals present (i.e. psychiatrists, nurses, psychologists, social workers, etc). Half of the community services have not provided any formal training for staff despite 43.4% of personnel having been transferred from public mental hospitals.

The shortfall in community psychiatric services is staggering and it is not just a question of the availability of beds, but also the development of sufficient community alternatives. What, however, can the inconsistency in service distribution and difficulties of implementation be attributed to?

Difficulties of implementation and subsequent considerations

When trying to clarify where the difficulties of implementation of Law 180 lie, one is immersed in a debate fundamental to how the reform is seen to function. From a macroeconomic viewpoint, the problem in the application of Law 180 is confounded by the way the budget for mental health care has been allocated. It is estimated that 80% of the expenditure given for mental health services goes towards maintaining the old mental hospitals. The remaining 20% thus needs to cover both the development and operation of alternative services. Calculating the overall budget allocated to psychiatric care, one finds that 8% of the total expenditure of the SSN goes towards this. The average percentage in Europe is 15% (Ongaro-Basaglia, 1987, cited in Mosher & Burti, 1989).

Mangen (1989) sees the problems of implementation in the structure of the Italian welfare state and the emergence of a fiscal crisis. He argues that many welfare policies, including those for mental health, "contain ambivalent and, indeed, conflicting goals so that varying interpretations of the task of implementation and the measurement of its success are inevitable" (p. 7). Regional autonomy in the organisation of health and welfare services, rather than improving efficiency in formulating policies, exacerbates the problems of implementation. The differing political orientations of each region also influence administrative procedures in the implementation of the reform. The fiscal crisis of the welfare state in Italy, the current status of the economy, and political instability – unemployment reaching 12.6% in 1987, increasing inflation at 15% during the economic recession in the late 1970s and the 1980s, and the submerged economy – have combined to heighten the difficulties further.

At the 'micro' level, a series of difficulties emerge in the way a service attempts to develop according to Law 180's intentions, if the hospital is still the central element in psychiatric services. One example (indicative of the majority of psychiatric services in Italy) is the mental health service in Trentino (north-east), based on intermediate structures. The difficulties are apparent where there is a worsening of care delivered and tension in the team's 'therapeutic atmosphere', exacerbated by the lack of formal training of psychiatric staff which has only seen a delayed or tentative introduction. This is further frustrated by the chronic problems of ward overcrowding, the inadequacy of interventions, and a lowering in the expectation of the reform's aims among patients and families.

Problems in the development of new psychiatric services are dramatically dependent upon the competence and style of work of consultant heads and individual local administrators, and this adds to the heterogeneity in service provision.

Still at the 'micro' level, some critics of the reform follow much the same lines as those who fear certain negative effects of the present trend in deinstitutionalisation policies. Ardent critics of Law 180 have expressed the risk of increased suicide rates, the possibility of 'wild dumping' and the abandonment of patients being discharged from mental hospitals (Jones & Poletti, 1985; Crepet, 1988; Crepet & Pirella, 1985). Contrary to these expectations, the number of suicides has not shown an apparent increase since 1978 (Tansella *et al*, 1987). Likewise, the number of those becoming homeless has not been identified in the post-reform decade (Bollini *et al*, 1988).

A further concern, often restated, refers to those patients in need of long-term care and whether facilities to meet their demands have been developed. It has been argued that the inadequacy in the formation and development of alternative services to the mental hospital has resulted in an extensive use of old people's homes and similar institutions (Crepet, 1988). The inability of district services to meet the need for long-term care has led to a moderate increase in the use of criminal psychiatric hospitals (Calvaruso *et al*, 1982; De Salvia, 1984).

A more recent issue is an increase in the less severe forms of mental disorder in the Italian population. Crepet (1990) points out that the sales of psychoactive drugs between 1981 and 1987 increased by 40.5% (Farmindustria, 1988, cited in Crepet, 1990). These forms of disorders are likely to occur outside the ambit of psychiatric services, implying, Crepet argues, a heavier demand on general practice and socio-health services. One indication of this is a study by Marino *et al* (1990) of both the psychiatric workload and the role of general practitioners (GPs) in the management of mental health needs in a population. Using the General Health Questionnaire (GHQ–30; Goldberg, 1978) on 505 attenders at 32 general practices on a specified day, they found 52% obtained high scores where the cut-off point was 5 or 6. With a higher cut-off point of 11 or 12 (C-GHQ) for long-standing psychological distress, 37% of the one-day population scored highly. The GPs identified 28% of attenders as 'cases'.

How have patients fared in places where a comprehensive community psychiatric service operates?

Case register data

From studies based on psychiatric case registers of the Lomest, South Verona and Portogruaro catchment areas, three main findings have emerged. The first verifies that community services have been put into practice. In 1984, Portogruaro treated 85% of its users in the community (Tansella & De Salvia, 1987). Using the same data, one finds that while admission rates to SPDCs have remained low and relatively constant, out-patient and day patient contact and domiciliary visits have shown a considerable increase in recent years.

The second finding from case register data of these northern areas is that there is little indication that 'new long-stay' in-patients are accumulating. A notable decrease in the number of in-patients has taken place, as many of these patients have now moved to long-term community psychiatric care following the reform (Balestrieri *et al*, 1987). In South Verona, long-term users' clinical and social characteristics have been found to be similar to those of the 'old long-stay' patients in mental hospitals (Mignolli *et al*, 1984).

The third finding is a substantial decrease in the number of compulsory admissions to SPDCs since 1978. The rate for South Verona in 1984 was 4.8 per 100 000. In Portogruaro during the same year, no involuntary admissions to SPDCs took place (Tansella & De Salvia, 1987).

Case register data for these areas appear to suggest that the implementation of the reform could be a success without the need to rely on mental hospitals, and emphasise the necessity of a comprehensive community psychiatric service.

Even where the reform has been implemented successfully, a pressing issue that continues to prevail is the impact on families of the mentally ill. How have families been affected?

Impact on the families of the mentally ill following Law 180

Families have been subject to quite serious neglect in the mass of research studies and descriptions of the post-reform era. This is surprising when, for example, one considers an area with an extensive community psychiatric service such as South Verona, where 83% of users are estimated to be living with families (Mosher & Burti, 1989), and are therefore in some way reliant upon them to provide much of the care and support. In evaluative studies of areas considered to have successfully applied the reform, little, if any, mention is made of families of users and it is still unclear how families are assisted and supported by services and staff, apart from through family therapy.

Family associations began to form in the early 1980s to express both their own needs, and those of their mentally distressed relatives. These associations fall under two main national networks: the Coordinating Committee for Mental Health (*Coordinamento Nazionale Salute Mentale*) and the Associations of Families, Users and Citizens (*Associazioni di Familari, Utenti e Cittadini*). The members of these associations are largely working women, mostly mothers and sisters of mentally ill relatives. Giannichedda (1989) outlines three of the objectives they propose. The first addresses the critical issue of the 'burden of care'. What families of these organisations propose is the relief of some of the burden (existing out-patient services and pharmacological inventions are not enough, especially with cut-backs in extramural services) by means of a community service open 24 hours a day, emphasising support and assistance for the material problems of the mentally ill. These two family networks differ in their opinions on the use of in-patient facilities. The

Coordinamento wants beds to be made available in CSMs and residential homes. The Associazioni, on the other hand, propose small or medium-sized wards for severe and long-term care as a means of guaranteeing a more consistent provision of care.

The second concerns the 'accusatory finger' often pointed towards families by mental health professionals. Often the family is viewed as being 'sick' or at fault in some way by some agencies; subsequently families are dealt with in an offhand manner, while staff are unaware of the disruption mental illness causes to the daily routine of families' lives. Such a viewpoint inevitably becomes counterproductive because the family may be providing most of the caring resources.

The third requirement is that services take on the responsibility for the mentally ill or share care with the family. Families also reject the passive role of caring for mentally ill members. It is not simply that families demand more information, rather they wish to play a more active role in the decisions professionals make. The suggestion of family committees overseeing the work carried out by mental health services has been put forward.

There is no doubt that the demands and opinions expressed by families are crucial to the way mental health services are to be restructured, particularly if they are to remain community-based. It is noteworthy that neither family organisation calls for the return of the mental hospital, although the fate of Italian psychiatric services and the reform surround this critical issue.

Future directions and conclusions

The problems of implementing Law 180 are now clear. It is now pertinent to ask what necessary changes are envisaged to make the system of community mental health care more homogeneous in its distribution across the nation and more effective in meeting the needs of the mentally distressed. What should Italian psychiatric care be aiming for now? Some, like Crepet (1988), say:

> "The innovations that have been achieved in Italy are fated to coexist with the old patterns of care and long out-dated scientific notions that are still preponderant in many parts of the country" (p. 522).

This stresses the lack of motivation to modify the 'old ways' of psychiatry that many practitioners wish to retain. Others, in their forecasts of prospects, are fierce in their criticism. A notable example is Kathleen Jones. In a 1988 publication she states:

> "The real lessons of the Italian Experience are that a law which is not backed by adequate finance and adequate training procedures to implement the

changes it requires is bad law. . . . It is unlikely that the money will be available either to make community care a reality or to build up the psychiatric hospitals again to an acceptable level'' (p. 68).

This point highlights a major difficulty. Most agree that the lack of financial resources and adequate training for staff are the source of many implementation difficulties. At present, attempts to remedy the limitations of Law 180 are producing an ongoing debate. A bill recently presented to parliament by the Independent Left attempts a 'definition, the finding and urgent creation of the services in the Department of Mental Health' and continues to strive for the phasing out of mental hospitals (Ongaro-Basaglia, 1989). Many other bills introduced to parliament with suggested amendments to Law 180 have focused on using beds in previous psychiatric institutions. Ongaro-Basaglia, however, argues that a more viable solution would be to create a model of mental health care based on a 24-hour service open seven days a week, covering the population in a given catchment area and providing full-time care for patients, if necessary, both day and night. Treatment would take place at home or in the surgery, there would be a provision of therapeutic residential facilities, and economic and social support would come from liaising social services. She stresses too that a mental health service of this type should not replicate the hospital structure because of the additional attachments of surgeries and social services.

The need for small residential units as an alternative to both hospitals and the family has been recognised. Ongaro-Basaglia maintains that this not only prevents chronicity, but gives families the opportunity to take on another role in support of their members – instead of being the sole carers bearing much of the responsibility, they are more involved in therapeutic plans.

This particular bill, encompassing all such proposals for change, has already reached the committee stage, aiming to create, in the short term, the necessary services. An additional law presented to parliament has sought to increase the proportion of the medical budget received by psychiatry to 8%.

What the future holds for mental health care in Italy is determined, crucially, not simply by the potential amendments to the reform act itself but also by the availability of financial resources allocated to mental health care and the willingness of regions to provide community mental health services. It is no longer useful to discuss only Italy's deinstitutionalisation or the current discharge of patients from psychiatric institutions; more pressing is how alternative community services are being developed across the country and the limitations imposed. Whether the system of psychiatric care in Italy will become more homogeneous or obtain the necessary expenditure to develop alternative services to the mental hospital remains uncertain. Yet it is important not to lose sight of the achievements of Basaglia, but to confront the difficulties and limitations that have emerged over the past decade with the aim of overcoming them.

Acknowledgements

Many thanks are due to Dr Ermanno Arreghini and Dr Ricardo Araya for their invaluable comments.

References

BALESTRIERI, M., MICCIOLO, R. & TANSELLA, M. (1987) Long-stay and long-term psychiatric patients in an area with a community-based system of care. A register follow-up study. *International Journal of Social Psychiatry*, **33**, 251–262.

BASAGLIA, F. (ed.) (1967) *L'Istituzione Negata: Rapporto da un Ospedale Psichiatrico*. Turin: Einaudi.

BOLLINI, P., RELCH, M. & MUSCETTOLA, G. (1988) Revision of the Italian psychiatric reform: north/south differences and future strategies. *Social Science and Medicine*, **27**, 1327–1335.

CALVARUSO, C., FRISANCO, R. & IZZO, S. (eds) (1982) *Indagine Censis-Ciseff sulla Attuazione della Riforma Psichiatrica e sul Destino dei Dimessi dagli O.P.* Roma: Edizioni Paoline.

CENSIS (Centro Studi Investimenti Sociali) (1984) *Le politiche psichiatriche regionali nel doporiforma e lo stato attuale dei servizi.* Roma: CENSIS.

—— (1985) *L'attuazione della riforma psichiatrica nel quardo delle politiche regionali e dell'offerta quantitativa e qualititativa dei servizi: Liguria, Mimeo.* Roma: CENSIS.

CREPET, P. (1988) The Italian mental health reform nine years on. *Acta Psychiatrica Scandinavica*, **77**, 515–523.

—— (1990). A transition period in psychiatric care in Italy ten years after the reform. *British Journal of Psychiatry*, **156**, 27–36.

—— & PIRELLA, A. (1985) The transformation of psychiatric care in Italy: methodological premises, current status, and future prospects. *International Journal of Mental Health*, **14**, 155–173.

DE GIROLAMO, G. (1989) Italian psychiatry and reform law: review of the international literature. *International Journal of Social Psychiatry*, **35**, 21–37.

DE SALVIA, D. (1984) Elementi di statistica ed epidemiologia sull'applicazione della 180. *Fogli di Informazione*, **106**, 1–22.

DONATI, P. (1985) Social welfare and social services in Italy since 1950. In *Social Policy in Western Europe and the USA: 1950–1980* (eds R. Girod, P. de Laubier & A. Gladstone). Basingstoke: Macmillan.

FARMINDUSTRIA (1988) *Indicatori farmaceutici.* Roma: Nuove Dimensioni.

GALLIO, G. & GIANNICHEDDA, M. G. (1982) Note per la lettura del modulo organizzativo dei servizi psichiatrici a Trieste. In *Psichiatria Senza Manicomio. Epidemiologia Critica della Riforma* (eds D. De Salvia, P. Crepet). Milano: Feltrinelli.

GIANNICHEDDA, M. G. (1989) "A normality for us without confinement for them": notes on the associations of families of the mentally ill. *International Journal of Social Psychiatry*, **35**, 62–70.

GOLDBERG, D. P. (1978) *Manual of the General Health Questionnaire.* London: NFER-Nelson.

GRIMOND, J. (1990) Awaiting an alternative: a survey of Italy. *Economist*, 26 May, 3–30.

ISTITUTO CENTRALE DI STATISTICA (ISTAT) *Annuario Statistico Italiano (1964–1987).* Roma: ISTAT.

JONES, K. (1988) *Experience in Mental Health: Community Care and Social Policy.* London: Sage.

—— & POLETTI, A. (1985) Understanding the Italian experience. *British Journal of Psychiatry*, **146**, 341–347.

MANGEN, S. (1989) The politics of reform: origins and enactment of the Italian experience. *International Journal of Social Psychiatry*, **35**, 7–19.

MARINO, S., BELLANTUONO, C. & TANSELLA, M. (1990) Psychiatric morbidity in general practice in Italy: a point-prevalence survey in a defined geographical area. *Social Psychiatry and Psychiatric Epidemiology*, **25**, 67–72.

MARTINI, P., CECCHINI, M., CORLITO, G., *et al* (1985) A model of a single comprehensive mental health service for a catchment area: a community alternative to hospitalization. *Acta Psychiatrica Scandinavica*, **71** (suppl 316), 95–120.

MARTINO, A. (1986) Italian lessons on the welfare state. *Economic Affairs*, June–July, 18–25.

MCCARTHY, M. (1985) Psychiatric care in Italy: Evidence and assertion. *Hospital and Health Services Review*. Nov. 278–280.

MIGNOLLI, G., FIORIO, R., FACCINCANI, C., *et al* (1984) Lungodegenza e lungoassistenza a Verona-Sud quattro anni dopo la riforma psichiatrica. *Rivista di Psichiatrica*, **19**, 97–114.

MISITI, R. (1985) Future developments in Italy. In *The Long-Term Treatment of Functional Psychoses* (ed. T. Helgason). Cambridge: Cambridge University Press.

MOSHER, L. R. (1982) Italy's revolutionary mental health law: an assessment. *American Journal of Psychiatry*, **139**, 199–203.

—— & BURTI, L. (1989) *Community Mental Health: Principles and Practice*. Norton: New York.

ONGARO-BASAGLIA, F. (1989) The psychiatric reform in Italy: summing up and looking ahead. *International Journal of Social Psychiatry*, **35**, 90–97.

—— and 10 co-sponsors (1987) Disegno di Legge: Provvedimenti per la programmazione, l'attuazione e il finanziamento dei servizi di salute mentale ad integrazione ed attuazione di quanto disposto dagli articoli f33, 34, 35 e 64 della legge 23 dicembre 1978, n.833. *Atti Parliamentari Senato della Repubblica*, **2312**.

PIRELLA, A. (1987) The implementation of the Italian psychiatric reform in a large conurbation. *International Journal of Social Psychiatry*, **33**, 119–131.

RAMON, S. (1985) The Italian psychiatric reform. In *Mental Health Care in the European Community* (ed. S. P. Mangen), pp. 170–203. London: Croom Helm.

ROBB, J. H. (1986) The Italian health services: slow revolution or permanent crisis. *Social Science and Medicine*, **22**, 619–627.

SCHEPHER-HUGHES, N. & LOVELL, A. (1986) Breaking the circuit of social control: lessons in public psychiatry from Italy and Franco Basaglia. *Social Science and Medicine*, **23**, 159–178.

TANSELLA, M. & DE SALVIA, D. (1987) Case registers in comprehensive community psychiatric service areas in Italy. In *Psychiatric Case Registers in Public Health. A Worldwide Inventory 1960–1985* (eds G. H. M. M. ten Horn, R. Giel, Gulbinat). Amsterdam: Elsevier.

——, ——, WILLIAMS, P. (1987) The Italian psychiatric reform: some quantitative evidence. *Social Psychiatry*, **22**, 37–48.

—— & WILLIAMS, P. (1987) The Italian experience and its implications. *Psychological Medicine*, **17**, 283–289.

TRANCHINA, P. (1979) *Norma e Antinorma*. Feltrinelli: Milano.

5 Spain: democracy followed by devolution

ENRIC DURAN and TOMAS BLANES

History and population

Spain consists of the mainland and the Balearic and Canary Islands; it has a total area of 504 782 km^2, including 12 287 km^2 in the islands (El País, 1990). The country's geography varies from the snowy peaks of the Pyrenees (north) and the Sierra Morena (south) to the desert-like areas in Almeria (south-east); from the green fields in the Atlantic (north-west) to the orange tree plantations and sandy beaches in the Mediterranean east or the olive groves in the south. The temperature on the coast is mild; the weather is wet on the Atlantic coast and dry on the Mediterranean. In the large central plateau the summers are hot and the winters cold. Andalucia in the south is warm and dry.

The population of Spain was around 39 million in 1986, 12.1% over 65 and 21.3% under 15. The population density was 77 inhabitants per square kilometre in 1987, the lowest in Western Europe (El País, 1990). The birth rate has gradually decreased during the last 20 years, in 1984 being 12.14 per 1000 population (Ministerio de Sanidad y Consumo, 1989b). Almost half of the population lives in towns of more than 100 000 inhabitants, and the concentration of population increases from south to north and from west to east. The most important cities are Madrid and Barcelona, each having a population of more than 1 700 000. During the 1960s people from the poor rural areas moved into large cities, the industrial north and north-west, tourist islands and other European countries, mainly France and Germany. This migration slowed down in the 1980s and has now nearly ceased.

Education is free and compulsory until the age of 16. In 1986, 3.9% of the population were still illiterate, but most of them were elderly people. Spain joined the EC in 1986. During recent years, economic growth has been remarkable. In 1987 the gross national product (GNP) was US $233 417 million – 12th in the world – with an income per capita of US $6010. Since 1984, the rate of inflation has been under 10% and in 1989 was 6.9%. Spain is mainly an agricultural country with industrial conglomerates in the Basque country and Catalonia. Tourism is one of the most important sources of wealth. In 1989, more than 50 million people visited the country, spending US $16 174 million. Most visitors come from other Western countries. Unemployment is the main problem in the Spanish economy. In 1985 nearly three million people were unemployed. During the last four years, this figure has tended to improve and in 1989 there were 2 522 000 unemployed, 17.3% of the active population (El País, 1990).

The Spanish Civil War (1936–39) resulted in 40 years of dictatorship which led to international isolation. When General Franco died in 1975 there was a period of political transition culminating in the general election in 1977. One year later the new constitution was promulgated and Spain became a parliamentary monarchy. The central government soon recognised the right of the historical nationalities to self-government. At present, Spain is made up of 17 self-governing regions (Fig. 5.1). As a result of these political changes, and the General Health Act of 1986, the Spanish National Health System (SNHS) is progressively being set up. The level of implementation in each Autonomic Region differs because decentralisation of power from central to regional governments is still ongoing. These reforms include the development of a comprehensive network of mental health services.

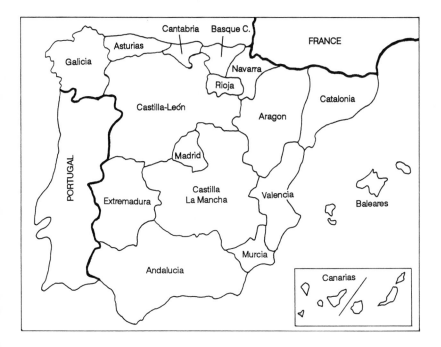

Fig. 5.1. The 17 regions of Spain

The Spanish national health system

Organisation and financing

The health services in Spain during the nineteenth and most of the twentieth century were organised in several independent systems and subsystems. They were poorly co-ordinated and often their functions were duplicated. The two most important networks of services were, firstly, those provided by the central government through the Social Security scheme created in 1942 and, secondly, those given by local and provincial authorities (Mansilla, 1984).

The Social Security scheme was financed on a tripartite basis by the State, employees and employers. The population covered by this system and the services provided were progressively increased over time. In 1986, 96% of the population was covered, representing about 37 million people, although variations between Autonomic Regions could be identified. At present, policy is to finance health services through general taxation and to cover 100% of the population. In spite of this high rate of coverage, a sizeable proportion of the population in some areas of Spain has additional forms of private insurance. For instance, a survey carried out in the city of Barcelona showed that 26.6% of the population have private and public insurance at the same time (Clos Matheu, 1989).

Local and provincial authorities provided a network of services for those without economic resources and not covered by the public insurance. In addition, they were concerned with public health programmes and with mental health services which were not provided by Social Security. These services were organised at provincial level.

The two systems were operated by different authorities. For instance, the principal authority responsible for Social Security was the Ministry of Labour, whereas local governments were the responsibility of the Directorate General of Health in the Home Office (Ministerio del Interior) (World Health Organization, 1981). Such a division of responsibilities led to a poorly co-ordinated and inefficient organisation of health services.

Coinciding with the first democratic government in 1977, for the first time a Ministry of Health and Consumer Affairs was established. Its main action was to initiate the reform of health services. The principles of reform were established by the Constitution of 1978 and can be divided into two key points. Firstly, the right of every person to free health care was recognised; secondly, the political organisation of the State would be based on 17 autonomous regions and the central government would steadily transfer power to the regions.

The political changes established by the Constitution, together with the problems in organisation and management of health services in the past, led to a long period of transition which resulted in the General Health Act of 1986. This act substantiated the basis of the new Spanish National Health System, which will be eventually composed of 17 Autonomous Health Services (AHS) (Fig. 5.2).

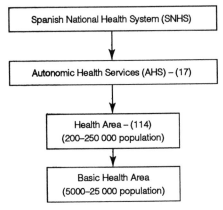

Fig. 5.2. Organisation levels of the SNHS

Autonomous Health Services will be responsible for organising, planning and financing health services in regions. In order to be effective, they will be divided into Health Areas each covering a population of 200 000–250 000 inhabitants. At present, Spain is divided into 114 Health Areas and each one will be further divided into basic health areas each covering a population of 5000–25 000 inhabitants (Ministerio de Sanidad y Consumo, 1989*a*).

At present, only six regions have promulgated legislation developing the structure of their AHS: these are Andalucia, Aragon, Galicia, Navarra, Valencia, and the Basque country. However, the management of health services has been transferred only to four regions: Andalucia, the Basque Country, Catalonia and Valencia. The remaining 13 regions are still managed by the central government.

Physical and human resources

The provision of health care in Spain has been organised on three levels: primary health care, specialised Social Security clinics and hospital services.

Until recent years, primary health care was provided to the majority of the population by Social Security clinics. Traditionally, general practitioners (GPs) and family paediatricians (FPs) worked isolated in these clinics on a part-time basis. They were paid by number of patients and were allowed to have their own private practices. A process of reform of primary care services has now begun. Primary Health Centres have been set up, incorporating full-time GPs, FPs, odontologists, nurses and social workers. Greater emphasis is placed on health promotion and prevention programmes and on the continuity of care, with specific programmes for chronic diseases. By 1986, around 400 centres had already been set up in Spain. However, there are regional and local differences in the level of development. For instance, the new system reaches about 20% of the population in Catalonia but only 5% in the city of Barcelona (Nebot & Villalbi, 1989). Because of primary health care reforms, specialised Social Security clinics are disappearing and becoming integrated with hospital out-patient clinics.

In 1986, there were 899 hospitals distributed throughout Spain, with a rate of 4.52 beds per 1000 population. There are five regions that have fewer than four beds per 1000 population, 11 that have between four and six, and finally two (Aragon and Navarra) that have more than six beds per 1000 population. Hospital services are about equally divided between the public sector and the private sector. Only 6% of the latter are non-profit-making institutions (Instituto Nacional de Estadística, 1989). In spite of the relevance of the private sector, a high proportion of it is financed by the public sector on a contractual basis.

In 1986, 13 296 medical doctors were registered at the Official College of Medical Doctors, i.e. 33.8 per 10 000 population. This rate, which is the highest within the countries of the Organization for Economic Cooperation and Development (OECD), contrasts with the still low number of nurses. The number of nurses in the SNHS in the same year was 143 773, i.e. 37.04 per 10 000 population (Ministerio de Sanidad y Consumo, 1989*b*).

Medical education

The high number of medical doctors can be explained by medical education policies during the 1970s. Medical education used to be open to any student who had passed the final school examination. The result of this open policy was an increasing number of unemployed graduates. Because of this situation and the need to co-ordinate medical doctors' training with health service needs, several reforms have been undertaken. The first step was the regulation of entry to the Faculty of Medicine. Since 1978, the number of medical students admitted has been gradually reduced and the number of

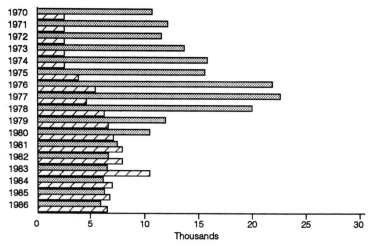

Fig. 5.3. Admitted (▨ *) and licensed (* ▨ *) doctors at the Spanish Faculty of Medicine*

places available is decided by the Ministry of Education in collaboration with the Ministry of Health. The impact of this policy is represented in Fig.' 5.3. As shown, the number of students admitted to medical school decreased from 22 554 in 1976 to 6166 in 1986 (Ministerio de Sanidad y Consumo, 1988).

The second step of the reform was the regulation of medical specialisation. The rate of medical specialists is the highest within Europe, 12 per 10 000 population (Ministerio de Sanidad y Consumo, 1984). In spite of this high rate, the number of doctors in each specialty was not consistent with the needs of the country. Now the number of places available every year is decided by an interministerial commission, according to the needs of the Spanish National Health System (SNHS) and with the participation of the Autonomic Authorities and the National Commission of Specialties. In 1978 two new specialties were introduced: Preventive Medicine and Public Health, and Community and Family Medicine. In contrast with the past, all institutions providing specialist training must now be accredited by the Ministry of Health. The training programme is based on the model of hospital residence. Since 1978, access to medical specialisation has been regulated by national examination. According to the marks obtained, doctors can choose what to specialise in and where. A study of the preferences of medical specialisation according to this system showed that Psychiatry is number 15 in the ranking (De la Fuente *et al*, 1988).

The medical specialisation policy followed since 1980 has changed the pattern of specialisation, the highest number of specialists being in Family and Community Medicine, which has increased by 63% since 1980. In 1980, only 38 graduates began psychiatric training, whereas in 1989 the number was 107, an increase of 182% (Fig. 5.4).

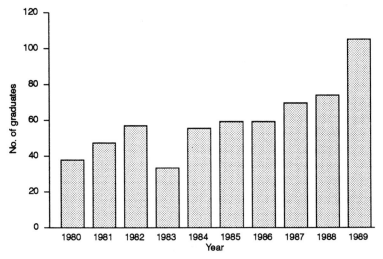

Fig. 5.4. Number of graduates beginning psychiatric training in Spain, 1980–1989

General health indicators

Health indicators in Spain show similar trends to other OECD countries. The general mortality is decreasing and life expectancy has increased from 35 years in 1900 to 75.6 years in 1980. Infant mortality was 9.87 per 1000 population in 1984. The general mortality rate was 820.5 per 100 000 population. The main causes of death are cardiovascular diseases (39.2%), cancer (25.1%), respiratory diseases (9.2%), digestive system diseases (5.7%) and accidents (5%) (Organization for Economic Cooperation and Development, 1987; Ministerio de Sanidad y Consumo, 1989c, 1990).

Mental health services in Spain

Mental health services in Spain, before the reforms undertaken during the 1980s, were exclusively based on large psychiatric hospitals. As in many other countries before reforms, asylums provided acute and chronic care to mentally ill patients. Mental health care needs were not recognised in the Social Security services. Local and provincial authorities were responsible for psychiatric care and developed most of the present network of psychiatric hospitals (Rodero, 1986).

Following the influence of other countries like France, the UK, the USA, Canada, the Scandinavian countries and Italy, Spain was looking for alternatives to this system. As a result of the influence of the thinking of Laing, Cooper and Basaglia, during the 1970s there was a movement mainly consisting of psychiatrists who criticised current psychiatric care (Aparicio, 1988). They pointed out, firstly, the poor living conditions and lost rights of mentally ill patients and, secondly, the lack of planning and shortage of appropriate therapeutic measures. This movement paved the way for the psychiatric reforms which began in the early 1980s.

The fundamental reform is the development of a new model of provision of mental health services across the country. This model is progressively being implemented at the same time that the SNHS is being reorganised. Although the national mental health policy was not established by the General Health Act until 1986, several government initiatives at provincial and regional levels started the reforms earlier. For instance, Barcelona (Catalonia) began in 1981 (Diputación de Barcelona, 1986), Asturias in 1983 (Garcia Gonzalez, 1988), Andalucia in 1984 (Instituto Andaluz de Salud Mental, 1988), Cantabria in 1985 (Rodero, 1985), and Castilla-León in 1986 (Consejeria de Bienestar Social, 1986).

Despite differences between regions, the most important problems were common throughout the country. These were:

(a) psychiatric care was spread out among different networks of services operated by the different authorities

(b) the structure of the services was inefficient and mainly based in psychiatric hospitals

(c) the very poor development of alternative therapeutic services based on community needs

(d) psychiatric information systems were poorly developed.

The most important aim of the reforms was to integrate all services under the SNHS and, based on geographical planning, develop a network of services according to community needs and modern treatments (Ministerio de Sanidad y Consumo, 1987; Departament de Sanitat i Seguretat Social, 1987; Consejeria de Salud, 1989).

Owing to the lack of information, it is impossible to present a detailed description of mental health services. However, the following strategy will be used to give an overall picture: firstly we describe mental health care levels proposed in the Psychiatric Reform, and secondly we explain the policy issues concerned with each level. Although it is impossible to generalise, we then consider some regional proposals as examples. According to the principles recommended by the Steering Group on Psychiatric Reform in 1983, and later established by the General Health Act of 1986, mental health care is being set up at four different levels: community, primary health care, psychiatric health care, and hospital psychiatric care which will be integrated in the corresponding health area (Fig. 5.5).

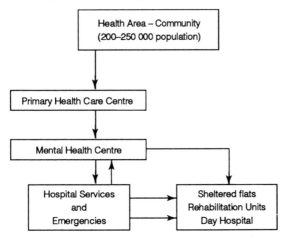

Fig. 5.5. Levels of organisation of mental health care within health areas

Psychiatry in primary health care

As mentioned earlier, the traditional general practitioner clinics are being progressively replaced by new Primary Health Care Centres. By 1995, the new specialty in Family and Community Medicine will be required by all doctors working in these centres (Ministerio de Sanidad y Consumo, 1990).

Although this reform started several years ago, few authors have evaluated its impact. For example, Villalbi *et al* (1988) carried out a study in a pilot centre which showed that hospital admissions and pharmaceutical expenditure have decreased, and that, in general, there is an improvement in the quality of primary health care (Rey & Villalbi, 1987).

This improvement should have an impact on mental health care. The Steering Group on Psychiatric Reform recommended several functions for primary health care teams. They should be able to identify psychiatric pathology and to treat and follow up the patients with psychiatric advice if required. They would also make referrals to the Mental Health Centres and be involved in mental health prevention programmes (Ministerio de Sanidad y Consumo, 1987, 1989*d*).

Although the necessity for co-operation between primary health care teams and mental health teams has been recognised, it is difficult to organise. Some authors have suggested that mental health units should be integrated in primary health centres (Albaiges & Isern Sitja, 1988; Isern Sitja, 1989). In spite of that, the present reform is setting up new mental health centres which liaise with, but are independent of, primary health care centres.

Mental health centres

Before the Psychiatric Reform, psychiatric out-patient clinics were reduced to private practice and to neuropsychiatry Social Security clinics. One study carried out in Andalucia showed that the latter dealt mainly with neurological problems (34%) (Instituto Andaluz de Salud Mental, 1988).

Although private care is still available, the neuropsychiatric clinics are disappearing and their professionals are being integrated with the new psychiatric services. The core of these services is the new Mental Health Centres, staffed by multidisciplinary teams. The number of professionals working in each team, and the number of centres, depends on the planning criteria of each region, although the disparity is not great. For example, in Andalucia, one mental health centre is being set up for each primary health care area. Staffing of these centres is as follows: one psychiatrist per 50 000 population, one psychologist per 100 000 population, one social worker per 100 000 population and one nurse per 75 000 population. One child psychiatry team per 500 000 population will be included in the Mental Health Centre. Andalucia in 1988 had 57 centres out of 67 planned.

Mental health teams should provide assessment, treatment, and follow-up for patients referred from primary health care teams and discharged from hospitals. They should co-ordinate mental health care at different levels, develop mental health promotion and prevention programmes, and participate in teaching and research.

Psychiatric hospital care

Because of the present reforms and the lack of up-to-date and accurate statistics, it is difficult to estimate the precise number of psychiatric hospitals presently operating in Spain. However, in 1986, according to Rodero there were 109 psychiatric hospitals with a total of 43 132 beds. This represents 1.37 beds per 1000 population. The psychiatric bed distribution by Autonomic Region is represented in Fig. 5.6. Although some general hospitals provided acute psychiatric beds, the majority of psychiatric beds were concentrated in psychiatric hospitals. According to national statistics, in 1986, 68.52% of the admissions were in hospitals owned by provincial governments and 31.4% were in private hospitals (Instituto Nacional de Estadística, 1989).

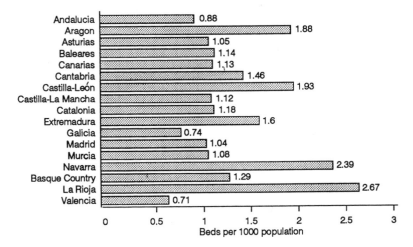

Fig. 5.6. Number of psychiatric beds per 1000 population by Autonomic region

The Psychiatric Reform has proposed a process of hospital deinstitutionalisation and the creation of new psychiatric units in general hospitals. After a careful study of the chronic population of the large psychiatric hospitals, different measures have been taken to achieve this goal. When it has been possible, patients have been returned to the community. When deinstitutionalisation is not successful the patient is transferred to mental handicap, psychogeriatric and psychiatric units, which are mainly located in the old psychiatric hospitals (Instituto Andaluz de Salud Mental, 1988).

In Andalucia, the new psychiatric units in general hospitals contain 15–20 beds. The professional staff consists of three psychiatrists, one psychologist, eight nurses and 15 nurse assistants. For the whole region, 22 units have been proposed, with a total of 515 beds. This represents a rate of eight beds per 100 000 population. Eight day-patient hospital units have also been planned (Instituto Andaluz de Salud Mental, 1988).

Psychiatric care in the community

Rehabilitation units and sheltered flats are being introduced at the community level. In Andalucia one rehabilitation unit is being set up for every 200 000–250 000 population. Each of these units is manned by a psychiatrist, a psychologist, a social worker, an occupational therapist and seven nurse assistants. Sheltered flats are being created according to the process of hospital deinstitutionalisation. In Catalonia, four sheltered places per 100 000 population have been planned (Departament de Sanitat i Seguretat Social, 1987, 1988).

In order to provide therapeutic and rehabilitation services for drug addiction, one therapeutic community is being set up for every 750 000 population (Instituto Andaluz de Salud Mental, 1988). Each one will be staffed by one psychiatrist, two psychologists, two nurses and about 12 nurse assistants. In 1986, there were 41 therapeutic communities (Ministerio de Sanidad y Consumo, 1989*b*).

Information systems and epidemiology

Information systems in Spain were reviewed by Gispert *et al* (1990), who found several gaps in mental health systems. There are only two periodic surveys that cover the whole country and provide data about mental health services. The first one provides information about hospital resources and activity (Encuesta de Establecimientos Sanitarios en Regimen de Internado). The second one (Encuesta de Morbilidad Hospitalaria; Instituto Nacional de Estadística, 1989) gives information about morbidity in the hospitals coded by ICD–9 (World Health Organization, 1978). Since 1977, when the health reforms started in Spain, some authors pointed out the relevance of the psychiatric epidemiology and the need to develop information systems able to provide data on the prevalence and incidence of mental disorders (Muñoz, 1981; Seva Diaz, 1982; Artundo, 1988; Fernando Arroyo, 1989). Therefore, some regions set up psychiatric registers and some studies were carried out (Garcia Gonzalez, 1988; Ten Horn & Pedreira Massa, 1988; Gispert *et al*, 1990).

The community of the valley of Baztan (Navarra) with 8575 inhabitants was studied by Vazquez-Baquero in 1975. The prevalence of mental disorders in the community was of 23.8%, being 19.2% for men and 28.3% for women. The prevalence of different disorders is shown in Fig. 5.7. The same author, using standardised instruments, the General Health Questionnaire (GHQ-60) and the PSE-ID, carried out a cross-sectional analysis of a rural community of the region of Cantabria where the prevalence of psychiatric disorders was 14.7% (8.1% for men and 20.6% for women) (Vazquez-Baquero, 1982, 1987). Finally, Herrera carried out a study in an area of Barcelona and found the same prevalence as Vazquez-Baquero in the valley of Baztan (Herrera *et al*, 1987).

In contrast with these studies limited to small communities that do not allow generalisation, the prevalence of drinking and smoking habits has been

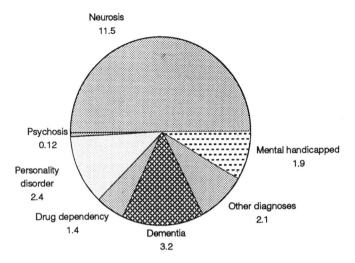

Neurosis
11.5

Psychosis
0.12

Personality
disorder
2.4

Drug dependency
1.4

Dementia
3.2

Other diagnoses
2.1

Mental handicapped
1.9

Fig. 5.7. Prevalence of mental disorders as percentage of the general population of the valley of Baztan

estimated for the whole country. The National Health Interview Survey indicates a prevalence of 38% smokers, 12% ex-smokers and 49% non-smokers; 30% of the population are non-drinkers, 10% drink occasionally, while 58% drink alcohol daily (Ministerio de Sanidad y Consumo, 1989*e*). The consumption of illegal drugs is an important public health problem. In 1984, a national programme for prevention, treatment and rehabilitation of drug addicts was established (Ministerio de Sanidad y Consumo, 1985). Because of the lack of data in 1987, a national information system on drug abuse was introduced (Roca & Antó, 1987). The mortality due to heroin overdose has increased since the end of the 1970s. During the period 1986–88, 655 people died because of heroin, 60% of the mortality arising in eight cities (Ministerio de Sanidad y Consumo, 1989*e*).

There are no population-based studies providing estimates of prevalence of mental disorders at the primary health care level. In a study carried out in a pilot centre in the city of Sabadell (Catalonia), only 6% of patients had mental disorders (Garcia *et al*, 1985). Padierna *et al* (1988) found a prevalence of 26.7%, but when the same medical doctors used the GHQ-28, the prevalence detected was 46.6%. A similar study done in the region of Andalucia showed that when the GHQ is used the prevalence is 42.7%, while when standardised methods are not used the prevalence is 18.61%.

Because of the recent creation of mental health centres, it is not possible to give population-based statistics at national level. In spite of this limitation, there is information on particular areas of Spain. Thus, the data coded by DSM–III (American Psychiatric Association, 1980) of 61 mental health centres of Catalonia showed that 33% of patients are diagnosed with psychosis and 33% with neurosis. Psychopharmacological treatment was

given to 24.5% and psychological treatment was undergone by 34.8%
(Diputación de Barcelona, 1986).

Mental health legislation

Spain does not have a mental health act. Legislation concerning psychiatric
admissions was included in Article 211 of the Civil Code, which was reviewed
and amended in 1983. There are two types of psychiatric admissions:
informal and compulsory. In the latter, a judge, after hearing the assessment
of a forensic doctor, will issue a court order to admit the patient to hospital.
However, in an emergency, the decision to admit the patient is taken only
by a doctor, who within the next 24 hours has to inform the court. Then
the judge and the forensic doctor should assess the patient to decide whether
or not the admission is appropriate. The judge should then collect
information about the progress of the patient and review the case at least
once every six months to decide whether the admission should continue.
The main problems of this legislation are: firstly, the right of the patient
to appeal is practically nil; secondly, social services are not involved in the
admission; thirdly, the forensic doctor is not specialised in psychiatry, and,
fourthly, the judges rarely assess the patients themselves.

Concluding remarks

In this chapter, the most important issues concerning the Spanish Psychiatric
Reform have been presented. However, as soon as this reform was undertaken, important problems arose. Thus, the implementation of the reform has
been very slow in some regions because of different political priorities of
regional budgets. Also, the creation of new mental health services has required
professionals who at the moment are not available in the country. Although
the number of psychiatrists in, training is gradually increasing, there are
still enormous deficits in the training of clinical psychologists, psychiatric
nurses, occupational therapists and social workers with a good knowledge of
mental health. Moreover, although mental health programmes of promotion
and prevention have been included as an important pillar of the reform, they
have not been initiated. Finally, the lack of information systems and research
teams makes evaluation of the progress of the reform very difficult.

As Spain in 1989 joined the World Health Organization programme
'Health for All by the Year 2000', it is believed that these problems of the
Psychiatric Reform will be partly resolved. The aims of this programme
in relation to the Psychiatric Reform can be summarised as follows:

(a) promotion of healthy lifestyles,
(b) enhancement of the information systems
(c) improvement of mental health manpower and services.

References

ALBAIGES, L. L. & ISERN SITJA, L. L. (1988) La integración de la salud mental en la asistencia primaria. *Atnación Primaria*, **5**, 68-73.

AMERICAN PSYCHIATRIC ASSOCIATION (1980) *Diagnostic and Statistical Manual of Mental Disorders (DSM-III)* (3rd edn). Washington, DC: APA.

APARICIO BASAURI, V. (1988) Apuntes sobre la Reforma Psiquiátrica. *Revista de la Asociación Española de Neurologia*, **VIII(26)**, 523-527.

ARTUNDO, C. (1988) Epidemiologia de Salud Mental. *Libro de ponencias de la VII Reunión de la Sociedad Española de Epidemiologia*. San Sebastián.

CLOS MATHEU, J. (1989) *La salut a Barcelona. Informe del Regidor de Salut Pública al Consell Plenari 1988*. Barcelona: Ajuntament de Barcelona.

CONSEJERIA DE BIENESTAR SOCIAL (1986) Asisténcia Psiquiátrica. Informe y recomendaciones del comité de expertos de Castilla y León en salud mental y asisténcia psiquiátrica. *Série Informes 6*. Junta de Castilla y León.

CONSEJERIA DE SALUD (1989) *Plan General de la Reforma Psiquiátrica de Madrid*. Madrid: Comunidad de Madrid.

DE LA FUENTE, L. *et al* (1988) La preferencia en la elección de las especialidades médicas en el período 1982-1987. *Gaceta Sanitaria*, **9**, 276-280.

DIPUTACIÓ DE BARCELONA (1986) *Informes Estadístics d'Administració Psiquiátrica 1986*. Barcelona: Diputació de Barcelona.

DIRECCIÓ GENERAL DE PLANIFICACIO I ORDENACIO SANITARIA (1987) L'asisténcia psiquiátrica i la salut mental a Catalunya. *Informes i Dictamens 10*. Barcelona: Departament de Sanitat i Seguretat Social.

EL PAÍS (1990) *Anuario El País*. Madrid: Ediciones El País.

FERNANDO ARROYO, M. (1989) Epidemiologia psiquiátrica: viejas y nuevas perspectivas. *Medicina Clínica (Barcelona)*, **92**, 269-275.

GARCIA GONZALEZ, J. (1988) La cuestión de la desinstitucionalización y de la reforma psiquiátrica en Asturias: cinco años de evolución 1983-1987. *Revista de la Asociación Española de Neurologia*, 8(27), 723-749.

——, APARICIO BASAURI, V. & EGUIAGARAY GARCIA, M. (1988) El registro de casos de los servicios de salud mental en Asturias: su implantación y utilización para la evolución asistencial. *Revista de Sanidad e Higiene Pública*, **62**, 1469-1482.

GARCIA PASCUAL, M., *et al* (1985) Estudio de los motivos de consulta por patologia mental en un centro de atención primaria. *Atención Primaria*, **2**, 24-28.

GISPERT, R., LESAGE, A. & BOYER, R. (1991) Los sistemas de información en salut mental: una puesta al dia. *Informaciones Psiquiátricas (Barcelona)*, **123**, 59-70.

HERRERA, R., *et al* (1987) Estudio epidemiológico en salud mental de la Comarca del Baix Llobregat. *Informaciones Psiquiátricas (Barcelona)*.

INSTITUTO ANDALUZ DE SALUD MENTAL (1988) *La Reforma Psiquiátrica en Andalucia 1984-1990*. Sevilla: Consejería de Salut y Servicios Sociales.

INSTITUTO NACIONAL DE ESTADISTICA (INE) (1989*a*) *Estadística de Establecimientos Sanitarios en Regimen de Internado. Año 1985*. Madrid: Instituto Nacional de Estadística.

—— (1989*b*) *Encuesta de Morbilidad Hospitalaria 1987*. Madrid: Instituto Nacional de Estadística.

ISERN SITJA, L. L. (1989) La salut mental i l'atanció primària. *Annals de Medicina (Barcelona)*, **75**, 173-174.

MANSILLA, P. P. (1984) Ley General de Sanidad. Conceptos básicos y principios generales. In *La Reforma Sanitaria en España a debate*. Madrid: Ministerio de Sanidad y Consumo.

MINISTERIO DE SANIDAD Y CONSUMO (1984) *Oferta y Demanda de Médicos en España. Una Primera Aproximación*. Madrid: Ministerio de Sanidad y Consumo.

—— (1987) *Comisión de Seguimiento de la Reforma Psiquiátrica*. Madrid: Ministerio de Sanidad y Consumo.

—— (1988) *Ministerial Consultation for Medical Education in Europe. Entrance, Licensed Doctors and Postgraduate Specialist Training in Spain. Facts and Figures 1969-1989*. Madrid: Ministerio de Sanidad y Consumo.

—— (1989*a*) *Ordenación Sanitaria del Territorio. Estudios Sanitarios*. Madrid: Ministerio de Sanidad y Consumo.

—— (1989*b*) *Memoria Estadística del Ministerio de Sanidad y Consumo 1986. Informatión Sanitaria y Epidemiología.* Madrid: Ministerio de Sanidad y Consumo.

—— (1989*c*) *Guia de Salud Mental en Atención Primaria de Salud.* Madrid: Ministerio de Sanidad y Consumo.

—— (1989*d*) *Estudio descriptivo de la mortalidad relacionado con el consumo de drogas en España para los años 1986–1988.* Madrid: Ministerio de Sanidad y Consumo.

—— (1989*e*) *Encuesta Nacional de Salud.* Madrid: Ministerio de Sanidad y Consumo.

—— (1990) *Estrategia de salud en el año 2000 en España.* Madrid: Ministerio de Sanidad y Consumo.

MUÑOZ, P. E. (1981) Epidemiologia y asisténcia psiquiátrica: la identificación de necesidades. *Actas Luso Españolas de Neurologia y Psiquiátria,* **9**, 283–302.

NEBOT, M. & VILLALBI, J. R. (1989) Health promotion through primary health care in Barcelona, Spain. A document presented at the Working Group on the Role of Primary care in Changing Lifestyles. Ravigo (Veneto, Italy).

ORGANIZATION FOR ECONOMIC COOPERATION AND DEVELOPMENT (OECD) (1987) Comparative analysis of OECD countries. *Social Policy Studies no. 4.* Paris: Organization for Economic Cooperation and Development.

PADIERNA, J. A. & COL. (1988) La morbilidad psiquiátrica en Atención Primaria: detección y derivación por el médico de familia. *Revista de la Asociación Española de Neurologia,* **8**(24), 21–29.

PROGRAMA DE SALUT MENTAL (1988) *Análisi i Propostes d'Acuació en Asisténcia Psiquiátrica d'Adults a Catalunya.* Barcelona: Departament de Sanitat i Seguretat Social.

PROGRAMA NACIONAL DE DROGODEPENDENCIAS (1985) *Plan Nacional de Drogas.* Madrid: Ministerio de Sanidad y Consumo.

REY, M. E. & VILLALBI, J. R. (1987) Impacto potencial de la reforma de la atención primaria sobre prescripción farmacéutica en España: la experiencia de Ciutat Badia. *Medicina Clinica (Barcelona),* **89**, 141–143.

ROCA, J. & ANTÓ, J. M. (1987) El Sistema Estatal de Información sobre Toxicomanias. *Comunidad y Drogas número 5/6.* Madrid: Ministerio de Sanidad y Consumo.

RODERO VICENTE, B. (1985) *Apuntes para un sistema de cuidados de salut mental para Cantabria: su desarrollo y aplicación entre los años 1985–1992.* Cantabria: Diputación Regional de Cantabria.

—— (1986) El actual momento psiquiátrico: perspectivas de futuro. *Revista de Sanidad e Higiene Publica,* **9**, 1201–1215.

SEVA DIAZ, A. (1982) Aplicación de la Epidemiologia a la planificación de la asisténcia Psiquiátrica. *Psiquis,* **3**, 174–185.

SUBDIRECCIÓN GENERAL DE INFORMACIÓN SANITARIA Y EPIDEMIOLOGIA (1989) *Memoria Estadística del Ministerio de Sanidad y Consumo 1986.* Madrid: Ministerio de Sanidad y Consumo.

TEN HORN, G. H. & PEDREIRA MASSA, J. L. (1988) Epidemiologia y registro de casos en salut mental infanto-juvenil. *Revista de la Asociación Española de Neurologia,* **8**(26), 373–389.

VAZQUEZ BAQUERO, J. L., MUÑOZ, P. E. & MADOZ, V. (1982) The influence of the process of urbanization on the prevalence of neurosis. *Acta Psychiatrica Scandinavica,* **65**, 161–170.

—— *et al* (1987) A community mental health survey in Cantabria. A general description of morbidity. *Psychological Medicine,* **17**, 227–241.

VILLALBI, J. R., AGUILERA, A. & FARRES, J. (1988) La utilización de los hospitales en España; efectos potenciales de la reforma de la atención primaria. *Medicina Clínica (Barcelona),* **91**, 761–763.

WORLD HEALTH ORGANIZATION (1978) *Mental Disorders. Glossary and Guide to their Classification in Accordance with the Ninth Revision of the International Classification of Diseases (ICD-9).* Geneva: WHO.

—— (1981) *Health Services in Europe. Volume 2: Country reviews and statistics.* Copenhagen: WHO, Regional Office for Europe.

6 The United Kingdom: breaking with tradition

LOUIS APPLEBY

In Britain, people are healthier and wealthier than in most parts of the world. Their children survive and live to old age, their water is clean, and they have enough food. Yet there is a health crisis. Once trumpeted as the peak of a long welfare tradition, the Health Service is undermined and overstretched and one of its priorities, mental health, is floundering. Psychotic patients live in prisons or sleep rough and a mass of morbidity goes undetected.

At the centre of the crisis is the present Government's plan to solve it, set out in a White Paper entitled "Working for Patients", published in January 1989 (Department of Health, 1989). In a hundred pages of proposals, two expressions rarely appear – public health and mental health. This chapter tries to envisage these vital areas in the future British Health Service.

A tradition of preventive action

Many of the pioneers of prevention who gave British medicine its colourful history made their discoveries with only a vague knowledge of aetiology. John Snow, always quoted by epidemiologists, knew nothing about *Vibrio cholerae* when he plotted on a map of Soho those houses affected by a cholera outbreak to discover that they were crowded around a water-pump in Broad Street. Yet his contribution to the prevention of cholera was not simply an astute observation, it was more importantly the intervention that followed it.

Edward Jenner, in what was arguably the key step in the most dramatic of all public health successes, did not even make his own observation. He borrowed from West Country folklore the idea that cowpox could protect against smallpox and then refined the theory until he was ready to experiment on a child from a local farm. The cause of smallpox remained unknown but its worldwide prevention had begun.

And so British medicine developed, through the great social reformers of the nineteenth century, like Chadwick and Shaftesbury, who eradicated infections, improved child health and prolonged life expectancy with a combination of social hygiene and employment laws. Preventive intervention improved the health of Britain's cities and industries by directing itself to populations at risk – children, the urban poor, and employees of high-morbidity industries. Thus the main causes of death and disease were defeated by focusing on population need rather than public demand.

Consequently, by the time the National Health Service (NHS) was founded in 1948, Britain was showing the low birth and death rates of today's developed countries. The birth rate was 18.1 per 1000 population and the crude (i.e. all ages) death rate was 10.9 per 1000 – both had fallen by 50% in 50 years. Infant mortality was 36.0 per 1000 live births, approximately one-quarter of the figure in 1900. Life expectancy at birth was 66 years for men, 71 years for women, compared with 40 and 42 years, respectively, a hundred years earlier, and 44 years and 48 years at the turn of the century (Office of Health Economics, 1987).

By the mid-1980s life expectancy had increased slightly, to 72 years for men and 78 years for women. But the age distribution had changed, although the total population had been fairly stable, and compared to less than 11% in 1948, the proportion over 65 was now above 15% and rising. The actual number of people over 75 was now 3.6 million, an increase of more than 100%. The crude death rate had not changed, but infant mortality had fallen to 9.1 per 1000 by 1987 (Office of Population Census and Surveys, 1987).

With and without the NHS, the overall changes have been towards fewer births, lower mortality in children of all ages, and a larger proportion of older people. The principal causes of death reflect these demographic changes. Circulatory diseases account for almost half of Britain's deaths, and malignant diseases for a further quarter. Ischaemic heart disease is the largest single cause of death in the UK; tumours of the respiratory system are the commonest fatal malignancy (Office of Population Censuses and Surveys, 1989).

Both epidemics can be effectively controlled only by preventive population measures, as both present to medical services at a relatively late stage in their natural history. Both have been convincingly related to environmental risk factors such as smoking which, because of health education and social fashion, has declined in prevalence from 45% in 1974 to 33% in 1986 (Central Statistical Office, 1989). As in the 19th century, the health services are preoccupied with treatment, but major falls in mortality must rely on social change.

This becomes more important if overall resources for health decline. Just as, according to George Orwell in *The Road to Wigan Pier*, when food is scarce people eat the least nutritious things because of their high energy content, so in the Health Service, when money is scarce it is spent on the things which least affect public health because they are more immediately pressing. So, medical and surgical emergencies have to be attended to, but general preventive programmes take second place or worse.

How the NHS is paid for is more complex than can be detailed here but there are two simple points to make, the first concerning comparisons between past and present funding. Since 1949 there has been a four fold increase in the cost of the NHS when calculated from 1949 prices. Yet, although NHS expenditure as a proportion of gross national product (GNP) has risen from 3.9% to around 6%, the UK now spends a smaller proportion of GNP on health than any other Western European country. The financial debate surrounding these contrasting yardsticks is complicated by arguments over inflation, capital expenditure, maintenance of facilities, cost of medical advances and changes in demography. But one further consideration is less often included, which is that the starting point for longitudinal comparisons, the initiation of the NHS, represents an already badly underfunded service, much too impoverished to cope with the ideal of matching health care to need. Against that background, the second point concerns the priorities of the NHS throughout its history. It has never been strong on preventive and public health because it has never been financially able to go beyond its more pressing acute duties.

In summary, health advances in the UK have depended on preventive public health, and to continue this exemplary tradition, two conditions are required. The first is a theoretical emphasis on preventive measures, with all that is then implied for medical education and joint programmes of health and social services. The second is sufficient resources to turn theory into practice after allowance is made for the needs of acute services.

Prevention and mental health

How can the public health tradition be continued to the advantage of mental health? Mental disorders make only a small contribution to national mortality statistics. In the UK, there are approximately 5000 suicides each year, less than 1% of total mortality. But within psychiatric populations, suicide is a substantial cause of death, and within society as a whole its pattern is changing as rates increase among teenagers and young men, and fall in those over 50.

Suicide can be viewed either from a pure public health perspective or as an outcome measure in the evaluation of psychiatric services, although the two tend to overlap. A full programme for suicide prevention would need to include the following factors.

(a) *Identification of risk factors and preventive influences in high-risk groups.* Although a large number of individual risk factors have been identified, Kreitman (1990) has pointed to the need for an integrated model incorporating both psychiatric and sociological factors.

(b) *Early detection of persons at risk.* Many suicides have made their intention clear to another person, often their general practitioner (GP). Early detection requires adequate education of health professionals and others in assessment of risk and in intervention.

(c) *Adequate preventive pathways.* Suicide prevention clearly needs more than the availability of psychiatric services. First, it needs a co-operative system of identification, treatment and referral in which primary care, voluntary agencies, casualty departments and mental health units in hospital and the community are linked. Secondly, it needs public awareness of what is immediately available. Adequate treatment methods include prompt management of depression and psychosis in primary care and psychiatry clinics, as well as facilities for emergency assessment and admission.

(d) *Suicide monitoring.* Obstetricians have the Confidential Enquiry into Maternal Deaths (Department of Health, 1990) as a triennial evaluation of their system of care. A similar monitoring of suicide would switch the emphasis of preventive research towards service use – and, equally important, lack of it – before death. No such national scheme exists. Regional schemes tend to be of two types: records of all suicides but with limited information on service use, and records of deaths after psychiatric contact but with limited numbers. Neither has sufficient information to suggest new interventions, and without new interventions evaluation is worthless.

Such a programme aligns itself firmly with one side of a public health dilemma. One approach to prevention in populations is to assume that lowering the mean value of a particular risk factor in a population will lower the risk among those whose risk is high. To quote the much-quoted example, lowering alcohol consumption in the population as a whole means shifting the distribution curve for alcohol intake to the left. The number of individuals at the far right of the curve is thus reduced and, as these are the people who may develop alcohol-related disorders, the rate of these disorders in the population drops. However, this approach works best when there is a powerful relationship between a factor and an outcome, as with alcohol and cirrhosis or smoking and lung cancer. Suicide is not related to its risk factors in such a direct way.

The other approach is to focus on those people considered to be at highest risk. For suicide, this means studying preventive factors in high-risk populations, e.g. recent psychiatric patients, and using what is discovered in future intervention.

In preventing psychiatric morbidity, the high-risk approach is the basis of tertiary prevention. For example, if poor housing is thought to contribute to chronic disability in psychiatric patients, there are two possible responses.

One is to campaign for better housing generally with the expectation that a general improvement will benefit psychiatric patients. The other is to seek better accommodation for the patient group only.

Needs assessment (Brewin *et al*, 1987) is the practical application of the high-risk approach, identifying likely areas of difficulty and disability in long-term patients and directing intervention accordingly. In another way too it is the continuation of the preventive tradition because here, more than anywhere else, the distinction between demand and need is most evident: the service needs of a population of psychiatric patients are potentially quite different from the competing demands of non-psychiatric patients.

In other respects, prevention of morbidity can be described under the same four headings as mortality:

(a) awareness of risk factors and their distribution in the population, e.g. hypertension for dementia, young children at home for depression
(b) early detection of acute illness, likely chronicity and long-term disability
(c) a clearly structured service integrating primary care and hospital units, with adequate clinical prevention, e.g. anti-hypertensive drugs, priority child care
(d) service evaluation leading to improved intervention.

If this is preventive psychiatry, how will it fare under the new National Health Service?

Working for patients

The White Paper, in outlining the so-called internal market, concentrates on financial and administrative reorganisation but believes this will re-shape the provision of services. Patients, it says, will be able to select the services they require and their health care will improve as a result. Staff who respond to ''local needs and preferences'' will be rewarded. Although not precise on the way these innovations will operate, the Paper does list seven key proposals, five of which are directly concerned with the practicalities of the market system.

(a) *Devolution of responsibilities.* Decisions on which services to provide will be made by District Health Authorities, but within prescribed limits. 'Core services' have been specified which must be made available by Districts to their local population; these core services include accident and emergency; immediate admissions, including to psychiatric wards; out-patient and ''other support services'' backing up the services already mentioned; and public health and community-based services including those for the mentally ill. However, it will not be necessary for a District to provide these services in a hospital within its own area, unless it is a matter of health policy that it should. It may instead buy them from a neighbouring District or a self-governing or private hospital.

(b) *Self-governing status.* Large hospitals will be able to apply to become NHS Hospital Trusts, earning revenue according to the sale of services to health authorities, GPs, private hospitals, insurance companies and other Hospital Trusts. The services provided will then be responsive to patient demand.

(c) *Movement of money across administrative boundaries.* This is the financial lubrication of the internal market, easing the movement of patients between one health authority and another and to private hospitals.

(d) *General practice budgets.* Large general practices will be able to apply for management of their own budgets with which they will buy hospital services for their patients. At the same time, GPs will compete for patients by offering the services patients want.

(e) *Medical audit.* Evaluation will be extended throughout the service, focusing on "quality of service and value for money".

The White Paper has not been short of critics but, viewed from a preventive mental health perspective, it makes some valuable points. It devolves responsibility for district service provision on to District Health Authorities who, in theory at least, should be most sensitive to the health requirements of their local populations. It then insists that Districts make certain sorts of health care available, the 'core services', and lists among these, acute psychiatric admissions, related out-patient care, community services for the mentally ill, and public health. It makes evaluation obligatory.

Nevertheless, it is flawed in at least three fundamental ways, which are outlined under separate headings below.

Need versus demand

In "Working for Patients" the terms 'need' and 'demand' are apparently interchangeable, yet they are quite obviously distinct, perhaps in psychiatry more than anywhere else. For a patient to translate need directly into demand he must recognise his dysfunction or risk, interpret it correctly and report it appropriately. Social disadvantage, lack of knowledge of health or health services and illness itself may impede the process. A homeless person with chronic schizophrenia may make no demand; a depressed mother may demand analgesics when she needs child care.

Need and demand may also differ qualitatively, as in the drug-dependent or alcohol-dependent patient who requests a particular type or duration of withdrawal. Furthermore, by their nature, preventive services will always emphasise need while patient demand is likely to emphasise acute care. The two are thus naturally in competition when resources are finite.

Cross-boundary referrals

The guarantee of access to selected core services for which Districts are to be responsible does not guarantee that the services themselves will be local. Because cash payments will follow patients across boundaries, the Conference of Royal Colleges which discussed the document believed there would be a "rapidly noticeable" increase in such referrals, adding to the work of the receiving Authority and depleting the resources of the referring Authority (Conference of the Medical Royal Colleges and their Faculties in the UK, 1989).

In mental health, the system will work against the development of an integrated service based in hospital, primary care and the community. It will be possible for a patient requiring a routine acute psychiatric admission to be referred to a different district or a private or NHS Trust Hospital and from there back to a community service unconnected with the preceding period as an in-patient. At a time when the social and health elements of community care are expected to integrate, this is a potentially fragmenting step.

Overall service planning

A successful devolved system would assess areas of maximum need at district level and provide the required services locally, while leaving less common or more complex needs for regional or supraregional services, set up as part of a regional or national plan. The White Paper does the opposite. It expects the internal market to create suitable services within and across districts. It creates a bottom-up system for referrals rather than a top-down system of provision. Consequently there is a risk of duplication, service gaps, and uneven quality and availability, made more likely by the special status of Trust Hospitals and the inherently patchy nature of private services.

The problems for preventive mental health services

It is easy to see how these flaws could undermine the components of a preventive mental health service.

Awareness of risk and its distribution within a population can be useful only if local services provide for a defined local population, which will not be the case under the internal market system. If, for example, different GPs choose to buy their obstetric care from different hospitals in and out of their district, a community-wide programme for preventing post-natal depression –

the commonest complication of pregnancy in the UK – will be severely hampered.

Early detection and prevention are aimed at high-risk individuals but, as with needs, high risks do not translate directly into high demand. Alcoholic women, for instance, do not seek regular liver function tests; drug-dependent or anorexic individuals are frequently undetected. There is also a degree of competition in the demand–risk divide. From the point of view of public health, waiting lists for hernia operations – singled out for action under the internal market – are unlikely to achieve high priority compared to depression in women because of the possible complications of depression, such as suicide, parasuicide, alcohol abuse, poor child care and marital disharmony. But prevention of depression and its sequelae will do badly in the internal market system because, when it comes to audit, depression is inconspicuous compared to a surgical waiting list.

Adequate preventive pathways depend on an integrated system of care. The internal market threatens to create a fragmented, incomplete and uneven system. In-patient, out-patient and community services will be divisible and different GPs in one locality may differ in where, and even whether, they refer their psychiatric cases. Public awareness of what is available, required at an early stage of the route to care, is made easier if that route is clear and, by implication, uniform.

The conclusion must be that a comprehensive public health approach to suicide, psychiatric illness and secondary impairment will be more difficult in the internal market because routes to care, and, therefore, prompt treatments, will be irregular.

Evaluation of all parts of the service is a welcome recommendation intended to improve quality of care. But what does quality of care mean? According to a King's Fund definition, it comprises six elements (Shaw, 1986):

Appropriateness – is the service what the population *needs*?

Equity – is there a fair share for *all the population*?

Accessibility – is the service compromised by undue limits of time or *distance*?

Effectiveness – does it achieve the intended benefit for the individual *and the population*?

Acceptability – does it satisfy the reasonable expectations of patients, providers and *community*?

Efficiency – are resources wasted on one service *to the detriment of another*?

The italics here are all mine, to emphasise a point. The internal market has been designed to make health care more acceptable to patients. Although it professes concern for each of the other elements of quality, its neglect of need and its market in patients may prevent it from improving any of them.

The way forward

To survive as a medical discipline, psychiatry must remain firmly within the NHS. To develop as a public health priority, it needs an NHS in which prevention is practised and financed. Britain has acquired and exported a tradition of health through public health which the NHS has been financially unable to cultivate and it is towards this goal that new policy should – and could still – be directed.

References

BREWIN, C.R., WING, J. K., MANGAN, S., *et al* (1987) Principles and practice of measuring needs in the long-term mentally ill. The MRC needs for care assessment. *Psychological Medicine*, **17**, 971–981.

CENTRAL STATISTICAL OFFICE (1989) *Regional Trends*. London: HMSO.

CONFERENCE OF THE MEDICAL ROYAL COLLEGES AND THEIR FACULTIES IN THE UK (1989) *Building on the White Paper: Some Suggestions and Safeguards*. London: Royal College of Physicians.

DEPARTMENT OF HEALTH (1989) *Working for Patients*. London: HMSO.

—— (1990) *Report on the Confidential Enquiries into Maternal Deaths*. London: HMSO.

KREITMAN, N. (1990) Recent issues in the epidemiological and public health aspects of parasuicide and suicide. In *The Public Health Impact of Mental Disorder* (eds D. Goldberg & D. Tantam). New York: Hogrefe and Huber.

OFFICE OF HEALTH ECONOMICS (1987) *Compendium of Health Statistics* (6th edn). London: OHE.

OFFICE OF POPULATION CENSUSES AND SURVEYS (1987) *Birth Statistics*. London: HMSO.

—— (1989) *Mortality: Cause*. London: HMSO.

SHAW, C. D. (1986) *Introducing Quality Assurance*. London: King's Fund Publishing Office.

III. Africa

7 The Somali people: refugees in two worlds

OMAR E. DIHOUD and ANTHONY J. PELOSI

The Somali Democratic Republic was formed in 1960 when the former British Somaliland Protectorate joined with the previously Italian-administered United Nations Trust Territory of Somalia.

The country occupies most of the Horn of Africa. It is bounded by the Gulf of Aden to the north, by the Indian Ocean to the east and south, by Kenya and Ethiopia to the west, and by the French-administered territory of the Afars and Issas to the north-west. It lies within tropical and subtropical zones and the coastal areas experience extremely hot weather. Parts of the north of the country are among the hottest areas in the world. Droughts are common, occurring every three to four years, with severe droughts every eight to ten years.

The population is around 7 000 000 and is increasing, with a projected doubling time of 23 years. In 1985, it was estimated that over 40% of the population were under 15. One-third of the population live in towns and cities and the remainder in rural areas, many of whom have a nomadic way of life which is dependent on livestock – sheep, goats and camels (World Bank, 1987; *Encyclopaedia Britannica*, 1990).

Political situation

The constitution provided for an elected parliament with universal adult suffrage; however, there was a military coup in 1969 led by General Muhammad Siyad Barrah. Since then there has been a military-dominated, single-party form of government.

The recent history of Somalia has been dominated by political upheavals. The boundaries established in 1960 have always been disputed and in 1977 and 1978 Somalia was at war with Ethiopia over the territory of the Ogaden. When the Somali forces withdrew, there was a high influx of refugees, mainly ethnic Somalis from the Ogaden, but there were other groups, including

Oromo peoples. There has been considerable dispute about these refugees and there are claims that they have been used by President Siyad Barrah's government to attack the local civilian population.

There has long been widespread dissatisfaction with the present government. There have been no multiparty elections since 1969. The human rights record of the government has been widely criticised (Ingham, 1990) and there have been claims that political opponents have been tortured (Amnesty International, 1984).

In 1988, the Ethiopian and Somali governments agreed to stop supporting resistance movements which were based in each other's countries. This led the Somali National Movement, which consists mainly of members of the Isaak tribe, to mount full-scale assaults on Burao and Hargeysa, the major cities of Northern Somalia, resulting in extensive bombardment of these cities by government forces. Hargeysa, previously the second largest city in the country, was essentially wiped out and it was estimated that 72 000 people died. The conflict created around 300 000 refugees in neighbouring countries and within the areas in the north under the control of the Somali National Movement; there was also an influx of refugees into Western countries.

Civil war has continued since 1988 in the north, and smouldering discontent in other areas has developed into full-scale civil war. The United Somali Congress (from the Central Region) and the Somali Patriotic Movement (from Upper Juba in the south) have led the rebellion in southern Somalia. Reports indicate that there have been widespread defections from the government army. In January 1991 heavy fighting in Mogadishu, the capital city, led to the withdrawal of foreign diplomats. At the time of writing, the government is attempting to reach a truce with the coalition of opposing forces. There have been recent press reports that President Siyad Barrah and his family are trying to flee the country.

Basic health indicators

The upheavals outlined above dominate the mental and physical health of the people of Somalia. The statistics presented here are those for 1987, before the outbreak of the present civil war. They are drawn from UNICEF figures (United Nations Children's Fund, 1989).

In 1987, the under-five mortality rate (the annual number of deaths of children under five years of age per 1000 live births) was 225. This means that Somalia has the 14th highest under-five mortality rate in the world. The infant mortality rate is 133 per 1000. The estimated maternal mortality rate was 1100 per 100 000 live births, which is the world's second highest. Only about 2% of births are attended by trained health personnel.

Half the urban population and 15% of the rural population are thought to have access to health services. In 1986 there were around 5500 hospital beds and 450 doctors (*Encyclopaedia Britannica*, 1990). This figure excludes personnel attached to refugee aid agencies. Green & Jamal (1987) have estimated that only 0.5% of the budget for development between 1977 and 1981 went to health services.

Psychiatric services in Somalia

Psychiatric services are probably the least developed of all the health services in Somalia. Most mental health interventions are provided as part of the general health care system.

There were three psychiatric institutions before the outbreak of the present civil war. Forlenini Hospital was built in Mogadishu in 1930 by the Italian colonial government. It has between 30 and 40 beds. The British built a psychiatric hospital in Berbera in 1940; this is known by the local people as '*Jail Magnoon*', which means jail for mad people. In Hargeysa, the General Group Hospital had a 30-bed psychiatric wing which was intended for non-aggressive patients. This hospital is no longer functioning, following the bombardment of Hargeysa.

It is not surprising that there are major problems within the psychiatric institutions. Although major tranquillisers are readily available, the lack of trained nursing staff means that physical restraint often has to be used. Electroconvulsive therapy, usually unmodified, is administered in Forlenini Hospital. The problems are at their worst in the '*Jail Magnoon*' in Berbera; no nurses are available and this has led to its being run by soldiers.

Traditional and religious healing also plays an important role in the treatment of psychiatric problems. These are sometimes led by religious leaders and can take the form of an exorcism of spirits which are thought to possess the disturbed person. At other times, healing rituals are carried out by women in the local community.

The refugee crisis and mental health

Political strife in the Horn of Africa has meant that Somalia has had the largest refugee population in Africa throughout the last decade. In 1980 over 1.2 million refugees were registered with the Somali government (Godfrey & Mursal, 1990); thus almost one in six of the inhabitants was a refugee.

A discussion of the implications of this for the Somali government, for its health policies, and for international aid agencies is beyond the scope of this contribution. Also, there are complicated political ramifications, and the need to take these into account when planning health interventions can only be acknowledged here. Such issues have been discussed in a broad context by Harrel-Bond (1985) and specifically with regard to refugees in Somalia in the late 1970s and 1980s by Godfrey & Mursal (1990).

There is scant information on mental health issues among refugees in Somalia. A report on refugee women and children in Somalia which focuses on their social and psychological needs has been prepared for UNICEF by Hancock (1988, unpublished).

Hancock conducted a questionnaire survey of 389 women and 778 children who were sampled from the inhabitants of 13 different refugee camps in four different regions. The survey has identified a wide range of social and psychological difficulties encountered by these women and children who had been in refugee camps for periods of up to 10 years.

Information on symptoms of emotional distress among the women was obtained using closed format questions on increased crying, nervousness, loneliness, and feelings of depression since coming to the camp. For example, the question on depression was as follows: "Since coming to live in the camp, do you become depressed more often?"

The table below shows some of the results.

TABLE 7.1
Symptoms of emotional distress in 389 women in refugee camps within Somalia

Symptom	Percentage showing symptom
Depressed more often	82
Nervous more often	93
Loneliness	83
Crying more often	71

The statistical data has been supplemented by case histories on 58 women and 23 children. These form a remarkable document which gives insight into the effects of past and ongoing catastrophic stressors and the variety of ways they have been dealt with. Hancock's experience led him to make a number of recommendations mainly aimed at lessening dependency and promoting self-sufficiency in these refugees. Also, he suggests ways in which serious psychological and behavioural difficulties can be detected and addressed by other family members and in school.

One of the present authors, Omar Dihoud, has visited refugee camps for Somalis in Ethiopia and can give anecdotal support to some of Hancock's findings and recommendations. Affective symptoms are understandably common, but at times they can be severe; cases of untreated psychotic depression have been encountered. Some refugees with mental health problems meet diagnostic criteria for post-traumatic stress disorder. Those with chronic psychotic illnesses are usually treated with chlorpromazine in high doses, although physical restraints are sometimes used.

Dihoud also found that the assessment of some of the most severe psychiatric disorders were complicated by head injuries sustained during fighting, and in some cases during torture.

Other problems identified during visits to the refugee camps included the overuse of khat, a stimulant plant which is used throughout East Africa (see Krikorian, 1984). This is usually used only sparingly but there is high consumption in the camps, especially by young men, with damaging effects on family life. Also, benzodiazepines can be bought over the counter and these are being abused, once again mainly by the young men.

The Somali counselling project in the UK

The Somali Counselling Project (Dihoud & Pelosi, 1989, 1990) was established in London's East End in December 1986 in response to the social problems and unmet health needs of refugees from the Horn of Africa who had come to the United Kingdom. The project was set up with the assistance of a grant from the City Parochial Foundation. Since November 1990 it has operated from larger premises in Central London.

Somali seafarers have been emigrating to the UK since the early 20th century and these ageing men now live in ports such as the East End of London, Liverpool, and Cardiff. Some moved to work in factories in the Midlands and there are Somali communities in Sheffield and Middlesbrough. The Somali Counselling Project offers assistance to these immigrants but most clients have been political refugees and asylum seekers who have come to the UK since 1980. Most are women and children, as in many cases the adult males of the families have been unable to leave Somalia. There was a large increase in refugees coming to the UK after the outbreak of civil war in 1988.

The work of the project

There are two members of staff: Omar Dihoud, and Ms Amina Hussein, a British-born woman of Somalian background, who is the administrative assistant and office manager. In addition, eight volunteer workers devote varying amounts of time to counselling and supporting clients. Further funding has recently been obtained which will permit the employment and training of an additional member of staff.

Currently, on average, three new clients per day consult staff with a range of social, personal and health difficulties. Most live in London but assistance is also given to people in other parts of the UK and occasionally to Somalis and culturally related peoples living in other European countries.

The project works with Social Services Departments, providing translation services, and advice on child care and physical and mental health issues. Because of language barriers, some Somalis are not fully aware of social benefits provision; the project frequently advises on statutory support and helps in the completion of claims.

We are often asked to intervene with the housing authorities. This may involve examination of housing rights and contact with Housing Departments to explain difficulties. Homelessness is a frequent reason for seeking help, and changes in the Social Security regulations in 1988 worsened this problem. Homelessness may arise in those who have gone to towns in the North of England but then feel isolated and return to London. We have a network of contacts with hostels (including church and refugee hostels) and with rental agencies in several parts of London.

Advice is given following marital breakdown, reasons for which include financial difficulties (often with poor management of money), isolation of the wives, and difficulties in acculturation. In our experience, women appear to bear the brunt of subsequent problems.

Mental and physical health

There is a high rate of physical illness and psychological distress in the Somali community. The many reasons for this include the stresses of migration, social isolation, economic deprivation and problems of acculturation (see Berry, 1988). Inadequate housing and a high rate of unemployment are additional serious problems. In certain areas, there is racial intolerance, the psychological sequelae of which have been described in other ethnic groups (see, for example, Fernando 1984; Littlewood & Lipsedge, 1988). However, many Somalis do not accept that they could be discriminated against on the grounds of race and this can make it more difficult to deal effectively with the problem. Also, cultural differences and language barriers often prevent effective use of mainstream health services.

Many have been subject to the unique stresses which can be encountered by political refugees. Their effects have been studied in clinical settings in several different groups of resettled refugees (see Miserez, 1988). Some clients have suffered imprisonment and torture. Family separations are frequent and there is often ongoing uncertainty about the fate of relatives in Africa. Many clients have suffered recent bereavements.

Communication difficulties leading to inadequate use of mainstream health services are a particular problem in mental illness and emotional disorders. One of Dihoud's main activities has been to provide a consultation service for general practitioners, hospitals, social workers and prison doctors. This involves advice on manifestations of certain mental illnesses and translation assistance. Attendance at psychiatric clinics and day centres is encouraged in those with more serious disorders. We are also involved in shared community care of psychiatrically ill clients.

Discussion of emotional difficulties in the clients' own language has been valuable and this is sometimes undertaken by volunteer workers under supervision. Anxiety management techniques are often suggested. Brief family counselling has been effective for some problems. At times, health has been improved simply by encouraging compliance with medication prescribed by family doctors or hospitals. Often, attention to social and immigration problems has led to improvement in mental state.

Some of these issues have been studied more formally in a pilot study of new attenders at the Somali Counselling Project. This study is described below.

Questionnaire study of adult clients

From October to December 1989, 59 clients were asked to complete a brief questionnaire assessment. The subjects were non-systematically (but not randomly) chosen from adults who had not previously consulted staff.

Assessment consisted of:

(a) a questionnaire in Somali on current social circumstances, in particular, employment, housing and family situations, and immigration status
(b) a Somali translation of the Self-Reporting Questionnaire (SRQ), a widely used instrument designed to elicit features of non-psychotic and psychotic emotional disturbance (Harding *et al*, 1980).

Results

The questionnaire was completed by 24 men and 35 women. Median age for the men was 30.5 years (range 17 to 56); the women's median age was 29 (range 18 to 66). Fifteen men were married, and 7 were single; of the women, 22 were married, 7 were single, 2 were divorced, 2 were separated, and 2 were widows. This information was missing for 2 men. Only one male and no females were in paid employment. There were three students among the younger clients.

Time spent in the UK ranged widely; some refugee clients had arrived in the UK less than a week before their attendance and others had been resident for many years. The median time in the UK was approximately four months. Forty-five clients (78%) had full refugee status; 8 (14%) had temporary admission status or were asylum seekers; 2 (3%) had exceptional leave to remain; 3 (5%) were residents. One client did not complete this section of the questionnaire.

Of the 56 who gave details, 34 (61%) were in bed-and-breakfast hotels, 7 (13%) lived in privately rented accommodation, and 15 (27%) were in local-authority housing.

Results of the self-reporting questionnaire

As expected, there was a high rate of non-psychotic emotional morbidity. The mean total score for the questions on non-psychotic emotional disturbance was eight (95% CI 5.5–10.5) for the men, and 11 (95% CI 9–13) for the women. The maximum possible score is 20.

A cut-off score of greater than or equal to eight, which indicates a high likelihood of having an emotional disorder of clinical severity, has been determined for this section of the SRQ (Mari & Williams, 1985). Using this cut-off score, 60% of the participants were probable 'cases'; 56% of the men and 69% of the women scored above the cut-off.

The questions screening for psychotic symptoms in the SRQ were considered unsatisfactory for use in this population. For example, the question attempting to assess the presence of paranoid symptoms is not appropriate for refugees. However, as expected, most (55%) did not score on this part of the questionnaire. Eight of the 59 clients scored 3 or 4 on this section. The significance of these positive responses is uncertain in the absence of further investigation; certainly, in only one client in this group was psychotic illness considered to be possibly present by Dihoud.

The small size of the study did not permit a full exploration of associations with non-psychotic emotional disturbance. However, some possible associations are worthy of comment.

  (a) There was a statistically significant higher mean level of non-psychotic symptoms in the women compared with the men (mean of 11 v. 8).
  (b) There was a trend to higher scores in asylum seekers or those with temporary admission status or exceptional leave to remain compared with those with full refugee status (mean score of 10.3 v. 9.3); however, this was a small difference which did not reach statistical significance.
  (c) There was no clear correlation between the length of time spent in the UK and score on the SRQ.
  (d) The mean SRQ scores were raised in those living in bed-and-breakfast hotels (mean = 11.2) compared with those living in private or council rented accommodation (mean = 7.5). This difference reached statistical significance ($P = 0.03$). Most of this difference arose from the male clients' scores. Among the men in rented accommodation, the mean score was 4.2; for those in bed-and-breakfast accommodation, the mean score was 10.8.

Discussion

The limitations of this study have to be borne in mind. The SRQ has not previously been used on Somali people and the authors have not yet been able to conduct a formal validation study. Some of the questions have been found to be misleading in Ethiopian subjects (Kortmann & Horn, 1988). However, the SRQ has been extensively used by other workers in a variety of settings (see, for example, Harding *et al*, 1980; Mari & Williams, 1985); we have found it useful in the day-to-day work of the Somali Counselling Project and the questions on non-psychotic symptoms provide for us a useful indicator of emotional morbidity. We are less satisfied with the section which attempts to assess the presence of psychotic symptoms; however, psychotic conditions are only rarely encountered in our clients.

The subjects investigated here cannot be considered representative of adult Somalis in London. They were all attenders at a counselling centre which includes in its aims the evaluation and treatment of psychological difficulties; therefore the high rates of such problems are not surprising.

This pilot investigation has confirmed the impressions of the workers in the Somali Counselling Project that a high rate of emotional morbidity accompanies the various social problems in their clients. In most cases the reasons given for attending were social problems rather than symptoms of emotional distress.

It was difficult to unravel further the associations with the emotional morbidity in this group. However, the higher rates in women are worthy of note. Also there was a striking difference in the symptoms in the men who lived in bed-and-breakfast hotels compared to those in rented accommodation. We were surprised that this difference did not also emerge clearly in the women. These findings will be the subject of further investigations.

Conclusions

The major political and economic problems which are currently being experienced in Somalia are having a profound effect on the mental health of the population of Somalia and on its refugees, including those who have been able to leave camps in Africa and obtain refugee status in a third country. Inevitably, mental health services will be inadequate in this situation. A resolution of the most serious political problems could permit the development of effective primary health care services in Somalia, of which mental health care would be an important part.

Acknowledgements

We thank the following for their financial support to the Somali Counselling Project: the London Borough Grants Scheme, the King's Fund, the Tudor Trust, Marks and Spencer plc, and the Allen Lane Foundation Trust. We especially wish to thank the City Parochial Foundation for its financial support and advice over the past five years. We also thank past and present members of the Management Committee of the Somali Counselling Project for their invaluable assistance.

References

AMNESTY INTERNATIONAL (1984) *Torture in the Eighties*. London: Amnesty International Publications.

BERRY, J. W. (1988) Acculturation and psychological adaptation among refugees. In *Refugees – the Trauma of Exile* (ed. D. Miserez). Dordrecht: Martinus Nijhoff.

DIHOUD, O. & PELOSI, A. J. (1989) The work of the Somali Counselling Project in the UK. *Psychiatric Bulletin*, **13**, 619–621.

—— & —— (1990) Mental health of Somali refugees in London attending a counselling centre. Paper no. 5.9. *Migration Medicine Seminar*. Geneva: International Organization for Migration.

ENCYCLOPAEDIA BRITANNICA (1990) *1990 Britannica Book of the Year*. Chicago: Encyclopaedia Britannica, Inc.

FERNANDO, S. (1984) Racism as a cause of depression. *International Journal of Social Psychiatry*, **30**, 41–49.

GODFREY, N. & MURSAL, H. M. (1990) International aid and national health policies for refugees: lessons from Somalia. *Journal of Refugee Studies*, **3**, 110–134.

GREEN, R. H. & JAMAL, V. (1987) *Paradoxes of private prosperity, poverty pockets, volatile vulnerability and public pauperisation*. A report to UNICEF, May–June 1987. Mogadishu/Geneva: United Nations Children's Fund.

HARDING, T. W., DE ARANGO, M. V., BALTAZAR, J., *et al* (1980) Mental disorders and primary health care: a study of their frequency and diagnosis in four developing countries. *Psychological Medicine*, **10**, 231–241.

HARREL-BOND, B. E. (1986) *Imposing Aid: Emergency Assistance to Refugees*. Oxford: Oxford University Press.

INGHAM, K. (1990) Somalia. In *1990 Britannica Book of the Year*. Chicago: Encyclopaedia Britannica, Inc.

KORTMANN, F. & HORN, S. T. (1988) Comprehension and motivation in responses to a psychiatric screening instrument. Validity of the SRQ in Ethiopia. *British Journal of Psychiatry*, **153**, 95–101.

KRIKORIAN, A. D. (1984) Kat and its use: an historical perspective. *Journal of Ethnopharmacology*, **12**, 115–178.

LITTLEWOOD, R. & LIPSEDGE, M. (1988) Psychiatric illness among British Afro-Caribbeans. *British Medical Journal*, **296**, 950–951.

MARI, J. J. & WILLIAMS, P. (1985) A comparison of the validity of two psychiatric screening questionnaires (GHQ-12 and SRQ-20) in Brazil using Relative Operating Characteristic (ROC) analysis. *Psychological Medicine*, **15**, 651–659.

MISEREZ, D. (1988) *Refugees – the Trauma of Exile*. Dordrecht: Martinus Nijhoff.

UNITED NATIONS CHILDREN'S FUND (1988) *The State of the World's Children*. Oxford: Oxford University Press.

WORLD BANK (1987) *Somalia agriculture sector survey. Main report and strategy. Report No. 6131-SO*. Washington, DC: World Bank.

8 Zimbabwe: fighting stigma and facing AIDS

SEKAI NHIWATIWA

Zimbabwe was colonised by the British at the turn of the 19th century, and was ruled by the British until 1965 when Ian Smith, the then Prime Minister, made a Unilateral Declaration of Independence, after which the country became isolated from the rest of the world, with the exception of South Africa. This independence meant more stringent apartheid and led to a bitter civil war lasting almost two decades. The war ended with black majority rule in 1980, following the Lancaster House talks which involved all the African parties, Ian Smith and representatives of the British Government, in September 1979. The talks lasted over six weeks and resulted in a cease-fire agreement. An interim government was set up, headed by Lord Soames, who led the war-distorted country finally to legitimate independence in April 1980. A general election was won by the Zanu Patriotic Front, which has since won on two more occasions.

Zimbabwe enjoys a more moderate climate than all the countries to the north of it. It is a landlocked country with South Africa on its southern border, Mozambique on its eastern border, Botswana to the south-west, Zambia to the north, and Malawi on the north-eastern border.

Zimbabwe, Zambia and Malawi used to be a federation of Southern Rhodesia, Northern Rhodesia and Nyasaland. The federal government headquarters and the university were in Southern Rhodesia, so after the breakup in 1963, Rhodesia gained a more advanced infrastructure and a more established university than its sister countries.

Zimbabwe, perhaps with the exception of Kenya, is the only multiracial society in independent Africa. The majority of the population are Africans from two tribes, the Shonas and the Ndebeles, making up 7.5 million. There are a quarter of a million whites, mostly of European origin, and half a million Asians.

The population of Zimbabwe can be divided into urban and rural dwellers. The majority of Africans are farmers by nature. It is usual for families to have their male members working in the cities and their female members working on small farms in the rural areas, although this picture is changing

91

rapidly as more women become educated and take up employment in the city. About 20–30% of Africans live in the cities while 70–80% live in the rural areas: the reverse is true of the white and Asian populations. Table 8.1 shows some of Zimbabwe's demography.

Zimbabwe is one of the most advanced countries in independent Africa, with well planned cities and towns, proper sewage plants and safe drinking water, and continued growth since independence. The main sources of revenue are agriculture, chrome, and steel, and, on a smaller scale, precious stones and gold. Coal is abundant, and it is now rumoured that oil has been detected.

TABLE 8.1
Demography of Zimbabwe

Demographic feature	
Population	8 250 000
Population under 15 years	50%
Population living in rural areas	77%
Population with safe drinking water	80%
Crude birth rate	49/1000
Crude death rate	15/1000
Annual national rate of population increase	3.1%
Life expectancy	
men	49–52
women	55–60
Infant mortality rate	
current	60/1000
at independence	120/1000
Childhood death rate (to 4 years)	$\approx 30/1000$
Maternal mortality	$\approx 150/10\ 000$

Health service

As Hollander (1986) has described, in 1980 the new Government inherited a centralised health service, organised along racial lines and orientated towards curative treatments. Despite this, it quickly adopted the World Health Organization (WHO, 1975) policy of health for all and accepted the components of primary care as priorities: health education, nutrition, water and sanitation, maternal and child health, immunisation, control of communicable diseases, basic curative care and essential drugs.

Differences between rural and urban health care remain, although they have been reduced. Rural clinics and hospitals are less well equipped and have less access to drugs. Rural communities are more likely to be exposed to unsafe water and poor sanitation.

Figure 8.1 shows the administrative structure of the health service. Below the single permanent secretary are several deputy secretaries who are

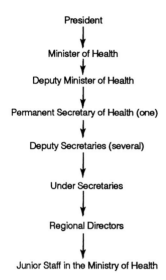

Fig. 8.1. The administrative structure of the health service

responsible for the various specialties, e.g. obstetrics and gynaecology, paediatrics, medicine, surgery, psychiatry, community or public health, pathology, pharmacology, personnel training, and health care planning.

Zimbabwe's health services are divided into two sectors – private and government. The general practitioners (GPs) are the cornerstone of the private sector (Fig. 8.2). They refer their clientele to consultants, most of whom also work in the government sector or are university lecturers. The consultants then admit patients to the private hospitals and private wards

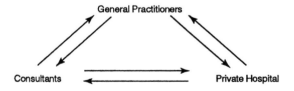

Fig. 8.2. The private sector

in the government hospitals. After discharge, the patients are sent back to their GPs for follow-up. Some of the GPs admit patients directly to the private hospitals and follow them through. All private patients pay; most of them are covered by health insurance schemes. All holders of medical insurance enjoy full coverage of medical expenses. Most GPs dispense their own drugs but a few give their patients prescriptions.

Figure 8.3 shows referrals in the government services. Referrals are made between different levels of the service. Basic care is delivered by the village

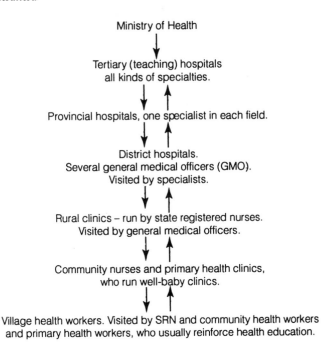

Ministry of Health

Tertiary (teaching) hospitals
all kinds of specialties.

Provincial hospitals, one specialist in each field.

District hospitals.
Several general medical officers (GMO).
Visited by specialists.

Rural clinics – run by state registered nurses.
Visited by general medical officers.

Community nurses and primary health clinics,
who run well-baby clinics.

Village health workers. Visited by SRN and community health workers
and primary health workers, who usually reinforce health education.

Fig. 8.3. Structure of government health services

health workers who have been recruited from villages themselves since independence and are well known to the communities they work in. They receive limited training for 6–12 months in health education and preventative medicine. They screen the villagers for infections and signs of malnutrition. Each village worker covers a distance of 5 kilometres.

The village clinics are manned by nurses, either SRN or medical assistants. They are situated at 10 kilometre intervals. From there patients may be referred to district general hospitals with 20-bed wards and day facilities, manned by government medical officers. After housemanship the GMOs go through three years of intensive training in all specialties so that they are able to treat most uncomplicated cases. The more difficult problems are referred to the provincial hospitals where there may be specialists and more surgical and diagnostic instruments. The most difficult cases are referred to the tertiary hospitals which are also teaching hospitals. Patients are followed up through the same levels of care but in reverse order. Zimbabwe has four major teaching hospitals in Harare and Bulawayo. The country is divided into eight provinces and each has at least one provincial hospital, two or more district hospitals and as many as 500 clinics.

Mental health services

Hollander (1986) listed seven mental health problems identified at independence:

(a) Negative popular attitudes to mental illness, leading to poor resource allocation
(b) Centralisation, leading to prolonged admissions in distant hospitals
(c) 'Mental illness' taken to refer to acute psychotic disturbance
(d) Lack of training in basic mental health for health personnel
(e) Lack of specialists in mental health
(f) Psychiatric management dominated by custodial care with little emphasis on rehabilitation
(g) An outdated mental health act, focusing on the process of legal detainment.

Thereafter, efforts were directed towards better education of health staff and the public, and decentralised, community-orientated services.

Mental illness

According to German (1987), psychiatric morbidity in black Africa is similar to that found in more developed countries. This seems likely to be equally true of Zimbabwe, although culture may colour the nature of the presentation. Delusions, for example, may be concerned with witchcraft (which is also a culturally acceptable belief at times). Schneiderian first-rank symptoms are also present, however. Many psychiatric patients are brought to hospital because of violence.

Most mildly depressed and anxious patients attend GPs before psychiatrists because they present with somatic complaints. Conversely, epilepsy is usually referred to psychiatrists, whether or not behavioural problems are present.

Drug abuse is rapidly increasing, and cannabis psychosis is common. Young cannabis users often grow their own cannabis in gardens or in the countryside. Other drugs are not common, except for barbiturates and benzodiazepines, and illicit drugs such as LSD and heroin.

Alcohol abuse and alcoholism are rampant in Zimbabwe. Drinking houses run by councils have been on the increase since independence, and the government receives a great deal of revenue through alcohol sales. There is a growing illegal network of alcohol sales, usually of native gin and toxic home-brews that rapidly damage the liver. Some users do not reach psychiatric services because they die before psychiatric complications develop. Delirium tremens is very common, often in accident victims deprived of their regular intake.

As in most African countries, infections and malnutrition may contribute to cases presenting to psychiatry. Cases of catatonia are still seen in Zimbabwe despite being almost non-existent in the West.

Human immunodeficiency virus (HIV) infection and acquired immuno-deficiency syndrome (AIDS) have become a serious problem since around 1985 when the first cases began to appear. There are many HIV-positive, apparently healthy carriers, and most are detected by screening when they donate blood. The proportion was about 23% in 1985 and has since risen to well over 50%. The number of officially reported cases was 119 in 1987, but this number is certain to be an underestimate. Deaths from AIDS are usually from secondary infections and Kaposi's sarcoma. The Department of Psychiatry had seen about 20 cases of AIDS dementia and many more of ARC (AIDS-related complex) by July 1989. The main modes of transmission are heterosexual, and much early infection was by blood transfusion. Several babies are born with congenital AIDS.

A committee set up by the World Health Organization to combat AIDS has embarked on extensive health education and practical measures such as the supply of condoms.

Projections for future psychiatric services

The infrastructure is already there (Ben Tovim, 1983; Buchan, 1986). What is desperately needed is more money to train personnel and make much-needed drugs more widely available. Extensive health education campaigns should be launched, to alert the populace to the danger of AIDS. Similarly, alcohol should not be promoted as healthy – instead its dangers should be made clear. Rehabilitation services need to be intensified so that the lives of the mentally ill can be as near normal as possible. Some work has been done already to try to destigmatise psychiatry through discussion in the mass media and organised interdisciplinary workshops, but more still needs to be done.

References

BEN TOVIM, A. (1983) Factors influencing integration of psychiatric care into primary health care in Botswana. *International Journal of Mental Health*, **12**, 107–123.
BUCHAN, T. (1986) Two decades of psychiatry in Zimbabwe, 1964–1984. *Psychiatric Bulletin*, **13**, 682–684.
GERMAN, A. (1987) Mental health in Africa. *British Journal of Psychiatry*, **151**, 435–439.
HOLLANDER, D. (1986) Zimbabwe: mental health. *Lancet*, **ii**, 212–213.
WHO (1975) *Organisation of Mental Health Services in Developing Countries: Technical Report 564*. Geneva: WHO.

IV. The Middle East

9 Saudi Arabia: acknowledging problems in a transitional culture

FAHAD SAUD ALYAHYA

The Kingdom of Saudi Arabia is located in south-west Asia, separated from Africa by the Red Sea. It occupies approximately four-fifths of the Arabian peninsula, an area of $2\,240\,000\,km^2$, but only 1% of this land is under cultivation. The climate is hot and dry. During the long summer months, midday temperatures may reach 48 °C. Winters are fairly cool and temperatures may fall to zero or below in the north and south-west. The average annual rainfall is five inches or less.

Reliable data on the total population are not available. Population estimates range from 3.2 million to 11 million, although six million is the accepted figure. The proportion of nomadic and semi-nomadic inhabitants lies between 15% and 33%. The majority of the population are Sunni Muslim, the Shiite minority being mainly in the Eastern Province. Seventy per cent of males and 81% of females are under 40 years old. The total number of live births in 1988 was 135 131 males and 128 828 females, according to birth registration. Oil production forms the main source of gross national product (GNP). However, development plans aim to encourage non-oil-producing sectors such as agriculture, industry and minerals. The state budget in 1988 was in the region of Saudi Riyal (SR) 140.636 billion (US $37.503 billion).

The total number of students in both general and higher education was around 2 million in 1984, 95 000 of these in higher education. Until recently, unemployment did not exist and there are no data regarding this new, but growing, problem.

Only a few decades ago, Saudi Arabia was a traditional, isolated, poor, and mostly nomadic country. Following tribal wars and battles with the Ottoman Empire, Saudi Arabia was formally consolidated in 1932 by Abdul Aziz Ibn Saud.

Saudi Arabia remains a monarchy. The King heads the government, and the council of ministers is the executive and administrative body. There is no constitution or parliament. Criminal and civil laws are derived from religious precepts, namely the Koran and Sharia Law. The Hijri Calendar, which is officially followed in Saudi Arabia, dates back to when the prophet Mohammed and his believers migrated to Medina in AD 622. A year consists of 12 lunar months and bears no relationship to the seasons.

Health services

The Ministry of Health (MOH) was set up in 1950 and is the main source of health services for the population. There are other governmental sectors, e.g. the Ministry of Defence, the National Guard, and the Universities, which provide health services for their personnel and for some other special cases. For example, Riyadh Armed Forces Hospital provides treatment for any patient with a malignant tumour.

The MOH is presided over by the Minister of Health. He has two deputies, one for executive affairs and the other for planning and development. Each of the latter has two deputy assistants. In executive affairs there is one for preventive medicine and another for curative medicine. In planning and development, the two assistants deal with development of manpower, planning and research. These four deputy assistants supervise 15 different departments of general administration (including a department of psychiatric and social health), which in turn supervise 33 different administrations (including psychiatry). Meanwhile 14 different health administrations are linked with these departments through the two deputy ministers. The private health sector is also supervised by the MOH.

TABLE 9.1
Increase in health resources since 1970 (national totals)

	Hospitals	Beds	Primary Care	Doctors	Nurses	Technicians
1970	47	7165	519	789	2253	1452
1985	105	20 796	1306	9257	20 707	10 086
1988	162	26 315	1477	11 940	27 169	14 013

TABLE 9.2
Non-MOH resources in Saudi Arabia, 1988

	Hospitals	Beds	Doctors	Nurses	Technicians
University hospitals	4	1421	889	2401	770
Armed forces	21	3635	1707	4088	2289
National Guard	2	722	486	1088	553
Security hospitals	1	116	372	565	284
Specialist hospitals	1	508	179	839	447
	1	175	52	195	52
Others	–	–	529	384	419
Private sector (hospitals)	55	5956	1890	5341	2071
Private dispensaries	–	–	2440	2253	1004

(There are also 592 private clinics, employing 666 doctors, 32 laboratories and 14 physiotherapy centres.)

All health services provided by the MOH are free to all citizens. The budget of the MOH for the year 1988–89 was SR 7.73 billion ($2.07 billion), which is 5.5% of the total national budget. Table 9.1 shows the increase in national health resources since 1970.

Less than 50% of Saudi doctors work in the MOH. This can be attributed to better management in the non-MOH government sectors, as well as better pay, housing schemes and educational opportunities. Table 9.2 shows the total non-MOH resources in Saudi Arabia in 1988.

Mental health services

The production of oil in 1938 in the newly consolidated Saudi Arabia started a new era for the country's mostly nomadic and tribal society. The process of building a modern state began and plans for massive urbanisation were drawn up. The sudden great wealth and modernity in a somewhat medieval society resulted in maximum development of the material aspect of life, but minimal and gradual change in people's thoughts and beliefs.

The majority of Saudis, especially in rural areas, attribute mental illnesses primarily to possession by demons – *'Jinn'*. The evil eye and, to a lesser extent, black magic – especially in cases of marital discord and psychosexual problems – are believed to cause mental illness. The traditional remedy is a mixture of herbal remedies, Koran verses, religious phrases and cauterisation. Often, the patient will be beaten up during exorcism.

The severely mentally ill have traditionally been isolated from society, and housed in various residences where they were kept tied up or handcuffed.

The first ever psychiatrist was recruited by the MOH in 1959 and was appointed to look after the residents of the famous madhouse in Tief. His main task at that time was to question the patients and to keep control.

In 1962, the first mental hospital in Saudi Arabia was set up. It was designed to accommodate 240 patients, but the actual number soon reached 600, and by 1982 the average in-patient number was 1138, while the number of psychiatrists was 32. The situation in the hospital did not differ much from that of its predecessor because of the overcrowding, poor staffing, and lack of proper psychiatric care and facilities. The hospital has been described as overcrowded, with much of the air of an old insane asylum (Dubovsky, 1983). By 1984, the psychiatric resources in Saudi Arabia were Tief Mental Health Hospital (TMHH) and a few out-patient clinics in general hospitals around Saudi Arabia whose main role was treating minor conditions and referring serious ones to TMHH.

Resources

The immense economic growth and the increasing availability of general health services has no parallel in the area of mental health. The crucial development in mental health services in the MOH took place in 1983 following a review of psychiatric services by the World Health Organization (WHO) and the reorganisation of the administrative structure at the MOH in the same year.

In 1983, the new hospital administration of TMHH quickly recognised the need to reduce the number of beds and improve the quality of care. In the same year, a psychiatric unit of 60 beds was opened in Riyadh Central Hospital. Almost one year later, this unit was separated to form Riyadh Mental Health Hospital (RMHH) with a capacity of 130 beds in six wards, and 14 out-patient clinics.

The Fourth Development Plan (1985–1990) emphasised the need to develop national programmes of mental health services. By the end of 1988 there were 14 mental health hospitals and four psychiatric units with a total of 1740 beds. There were also 15 out-patient clinics in general hospitals.

There are currently two Amal hospitals in Riyadh and Damman, each with 280 beds, designed to treat alcoholics and drug addicts only. These beds raise the total number to 2120. A third Amal hospital is currently under construction in Jeddah.

The total number of psychiatrists working for the MOH is 148 (of whom 16 are Saudis). There are 57 social workers working at MOH mental hospitals and units, but the national total, including those who work in general wards, is 235. There are 70 psychologists in the Kingdom, but it is not clear how many of these are clinical psychologists. Apart from MOH facilities, other government sectors, including Armed Forces Hospitals, National Guard Hospitals, and University Hospitals, have 102 psychiatric beds and 52 psychiatrists. The private sector has 180 psychiatric beds and 37 full-time psychiatrists as well as five private clinics with five psychiatrists. The total number of psychiatrists in Saudi Arabia in 1989 was 242.

Training

A two-year diploma course in psychiatry was started at TMHH in 1976, with supervision from King Saud University in Riyadh, but it was discontinued in 1983, after 29 psychiatrists had received it, because it was not recognised outside Saudi Arabia. Currently, two of the four existing faculties in Saudi Arabia award a diploma in psychiatry, although the number of doctors who enrol is small. In 1989, six psychiatrists were awarded the diploma at King Khalid University Hospital in Riyadh.

While there are 31 health institutes (16 for males and 15 for females) for the training of nurses and paramedical staff, none of them offers a specific psychiatric programme. However, a diploma in psychiatry will soon be established. There are several faculties of education with hundreds of psychology students in Saudi Arabia. There were, however, no provisions for clinical psychology training until 1989 when King Saud University in Riyadh started a division of clinical psychology. Students are also sent abroad to obtain training in psychiatry or clinical psychology. Although this continues, it has been affected by the reduction in government budget and the fall in oil prices.

Research

Unfortunately, Saudi Arabia is lacking in epidemiological studies, which are essential for planning and maintaining any psychiatric services. There are no reliable objective data regarding prevalence and incidence. The only information source, medical records, is not capable of providing accurate data. The MOH report on medical research for 1989 did not include any psychiatric research project. However, plans for psychiatric research and epidemiological studies have been recognised as an urgent need.

Because of poor information, contradictory findings are to be expected. An RMHH report has stated anxiety, depression and paranoia to be the most frequently seen conditions. TMHH statistics show that 57.5% of in-patients in 1983 were schizophrenic, 13% mentally retarded, and 29% 'others'. This can be explained by the fact that TMHH is the only hospital in the Kingdom which is prepared to accommodate chronic severely ill patients.

Analysis of several statistical accounts suggest that, per 1000 population, 10–20 suffer from severe mental illness, 40–50 have neurotic and emotional disorders, 20 have some sort of mental retardation, and 5 suffer from epilepsy. The prevalence of senile dementia in individuals aged 70 years or more is 100–200 per 1000. Chronic schizophrenics who need long-term care, rehabilitation, and reintegrating into the community number 5 per 1000 persons.

From MOH reports, the total number of admissions through its psychiatric facilities was 8984 in 1988, and the total number of out-patients seen throughout the country in the same year was 364 648. Overall, the mental disorders were as follows:

Neurotic disorders	40%
Psychotic	17.1%
Alcoholics and drug addicts	17%
Epilepsy	0.2%
Mental retardation	3.3%
Others	7.2%
Referred for psychiatric assessment for the eligibility to carry weapons, hold a driving licence, etc.	9%

Data obtained from social work studies of general hospital patients in 1988 showed that 23% had psychological problems related to their physical illness, 5.6% had family problems, 2.8% had occupational problems and 7.4% were handicapped. In other words, about 40% of 25 887 patients in general wards had some form of psychological problem.

Conversion hysteria is not an uncommon condition in Saudi Arabia. Suicide attempts are seldom reported, as Islam prohibits suicide, and suicidal patients rarely express these thoughts. There is no available record of suicide, but Riyadh Central Hospital records more than 400 suicide attempts each year. Possible police involvement must lessen the likelihood of reporting.

Until recently, alcohol and drug problems were denied – the official figure for alcoholism was close to zero – because of the legal prohibitions against alcohol. It was feared that admitting the existence of such a problem would embarrass the country as the leader of Muslim nations. This unrealistic denial was replaced almost three years ago by a full recognition of the problem, followed by the setting up of specialised hospitals for addicts and alcoholics and of treatment facilities in other mental health institutions, and the dropping of legal charges against those who seek help. However, there are severe punishments for dealers and distributors.

Mental health legislation

There is no mental health legislation. An enormous effort to create a mental health act was aborted in 1988 because of administrative difficulties in the MOH. Sharia law provides for diminished responsibility for the mentally unfit, but rules are still vague and differ from one psychiatrist to another. Compulsory admission and treatments have not yet been addressed. Pasnue & Hortmann (1983) emphasised the importance of finding a way to develop new legal guidelines in the context of traditional Islamic law and custom.

Towards the Year 2000

As Saudi Arabia is a signatory of the Alma-Ata Declaration (1977), Saudi national strategies have been developed to meet the challenge, ''Health For All by the Year 2000''. Unfortunately, mental health was not included and efforts are urgently needed to correct this omission.

In 1977, there was one psychiatrist for every two million people, in 1983 this figure was improved to 1 per 200 000 population, and in 1988 it showed further improvement to 1.2 per 100 000 people. Yet, this ratio is far from the minimum ratio stipulated by the WHO, i.e. one psychiatrist per 8000 population.

The National Mental Health programme aims to get much closer to the WHO recommendations. Several strategies have been proposed: integrating mental health services through primary health care centres, promotion of mental health facilities, training, and co-operation with non-health sectors. The main idea is to incorporate mental health within primary health care (PHC) centres staffed by social workers and/or psychologists in addition to the PHC team. Mental health professionals will train and supervise the medical personnel who form the treatment team. The main task of PHC will be case identification, counselling, and treatment of minor conditions. Through

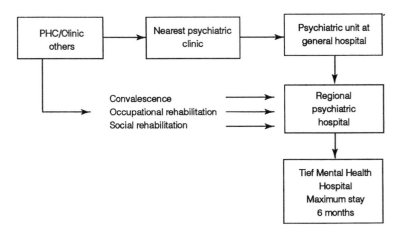

Fig. 9.1. Progress of Mental Health Services in Saudi Arabia – MOH

a series of referral systems, the PHC will be linked with mental health services. Figure 9.1 shows the relationship between the PHC and the mental health services.

To encourage recruitment in mental health facilities, a monthly bonus is offered, ranging from 30–100% of basic salaries according to profession and post.

The challenges facing Saudi psychiatry

Social change

There have been important economic and social changes in Saudi Arabia, affecting all aspects of life. An aggressive drive towards modernisation and urbanisation has occurred, while traditional values have been maintained, and this has led to problems frequently seen during rapid urbanisation. However, in such a strict, traditional society, the conflict between the old and the new has reached all sorts of activities. Personal insecurity and instability and neurotic problems are expected to peak. The transformation from extended to nuclear families is leading to family and marital problems and limiting social support networks.

Another important aspect of this transition lies in the situation of Saudi women. There is a growing conflict between the traditional female role – to marry and bear children – and the newly developed image of working women. The opportunity to gain education and to travel has led to an awareness in women of their situation in a strict society where, for instance, they are not permitted to drive. This conflict may be significant in the development of psychosocial and neurotic problems. On the other hand, psychiatric records, while showing an increase in female patients, still show a female:male ratio of 1:3. This paradox is due to the fact that women do not have easy access to psychiatric help. Often a female patient will be brought to a psychiatric centre only when she is extremely disturbed or disinhibited and her family is failing to cope with her. Utilisation of community-based psychiatry and home visits by properly trained personnel are essential in the assessment, treatment and prevention of psychiatric morbidity in females.

A third consequence deserves special mention, the growing alcohol- and drug-related problems in Saudi. There are two important facts to note. Firstly, these problems are international, and global attention has recently been drawn to them by international organisations. Secondly, the economic and social changes in Saudi have included migration to cities, travelling abroad in huge numbers, recruitment of foreign workers, and mixing with other communities either domestically or abroad. Young people form a large proportion of these travellers and they are more likely to acquire alcohol- and drug-related problems. This could explain to some extent the recent rise in alcoholics and drug addicts in Saudi but another consideration is the current lifestyle of young Saudis. The dramatic modernisation in Saudi Arabia has put extra pressure on these people, and together with social and family oppression, frustration, and lack of sport and social facilities, conflict between individuality and traditional norms leads to the abuse of alcohol and drugs. The National Mental Health Programme suggests several measures such as counselling, guidance, and education, but does not refer to the lack of leisure opportunities.

Professional disputes

Administration is a serious problem in developing countries. In the early 1970s, Saudi Arabia adopted a plan for 'Saudization', which implies the replacement of non-Saudis in administration by qualified Saudis, a valid and constructive notion if it is followed properly and gradually. The plan reached psychiatry in the first half of the 1980s, when an aggressive plan to promote and develop psychiatric services was set up. As a result, the psychologists, who were – and still are – much more numerous than the psychiatrists (in 1988 there were 16 Saudi psychiatrists working at MOH compared with 70 Saudi psychologists), received the majority of administrative posts either at clinic level or higher. The vast majority of those psychologists were educational or social psychologists and little administrative or clinical background was the norm. This has led to several problems: absence of proper teamwork, restriction of drug prescription by psychiatrists to three or seven days, unless permission is obtained from the clinic manager (a psychologist), and growing tension between the members of the treatment team. In 1984 electroconvulsive therapy (ECT) was totally prohibited by the administrator of TMHH, but it was reintroduced several months later. Although the restrictions imposed on drugs and ECT can be partly understood as a reaction to their previous abuse, both in private and public psychiatric facilities, there is no justification for severe restrictions or for complete abandonment.

The definition of psychiatrist and psychologist at the General Administration of Social and Mental Health (GAMSH) at MOH is vague and controversial. Official literature seldom distinguishes between a clinical psychologist and other psychologists. Definitions adopted are:

> "The psychiatrist is a doctor specialised in symptoms that the patient complains from as well as his relatives' accounts, and by aids of medical and social reports he will examine all contributing factors in the psychiatric case, and accordingly he will provide a preliminary diagnosis and will prescribe the proper medication. . . ."

> "The psychologist is a person who is specialised in the diagnosis and treatment of psychiatric diseases, providing psychotherapy sessions and utilising different schools of psychotherapy, psychoanalysis, behavioural and humanitarian. . . ."

Education

There are currently four medical schools in Saudi Arabia. Although teaching is of a high standard, psychiatric teaching for undergraduates is restricted to a few lectures on basic topics such as depression and organic brain syndromes. Human behaviour, psychopathology and other basic science courses in psychiatry are not offered. There is obviously an urgent need to correct the medical curriculum to include proper basic psychiatric teaching. Less obvious is the need for intensive courses, lectures, case conferences and seminars for non-psychiatric doctors and paramedics.

Diagnosis and classification

A scheme of classification and diagnosis of mental illnesses is still unavailable in Saudi Arabia, even though the country has officially adopted the ICD-9 (World Health Organization, 1978). This matter is still individual and optional, and psychiatric departments or even psychiatrists follow any scheme that suits them. For instance, the psychiatric unit at the Armed Forces Hospital in Riyadh follows the ICD-9, while the DSM-III (American Psychiatric Association, 1980) is used by both psychiatric clinics in the National Guard Hospital and King Faisal Specialist Hospital in Riyadh. On the other hand, a psychiatrist at MOH centres will follow the scheme adopted by him according to his nationality and the country he was trained in. This discrepancy in diagnostic approaches limits the use of medical records as sources of information and reduces proper communication between psychiatrists throughout Saudi.

Psychotherapy

It is worth emphasising the need for modified psychotherapeutic approaches appropriate to the need, culture and traditions of Saudi Arabia. Antipsychotic drugs and religious exhortation have been used much more frequently than milieu therapies, and biopsychosocial approaches are now needed as well as other scientific remedies.

The Arab Board in Psychiatry stipulates four years' experience in recognised hospitals, including one year in psychotherapy. Moreover, candidates are expected to carry out a study or thesis in psychotherapy.

Public awareness

Analysis of the available statistics and data revealed sharp increases in the total numbers attending psychiatric facilities. This apparent increase may be related to both dissemination of mental health facilities and growing mental health awareness. Yet the old notions of *jinn*, the evil eye and black magic are still prevalent among large sectors of the population, and, accordingly, people seek the help of traditional healers rather than professionals. The utilisation of mass media could therefore be of great value in the promotion of mental health awareness.

Traditional healers

The traditional belief system and the increase in rates of psychiatric morbidity ensure brisk business for traditional healers. Patients, by seeking the help of traditional healers, avoid the stigma of being psychiatric patients, and also receive an explanation consistent with their beliefs. Unfortunately, only some of the cases with which the psychiatrists have failed are cured by the traditional healers; others are made much worse.

Healers could play an important role in the Saudi psychiatric services but it is essential that roles are first defined and that their activities are governed by an authorised and recognised organisation.

References

AMERICAN PSYCHIATRIC ASSOCIATION (1980) *Diagnostic and Statistical Manual of Mental Disorders* (3rd edn) (DSM–III). Washington, DC: APA.
DUBOVSKY, S. L. (1983) Psychiatry in Saudi Arabia. *American Journal of Psychiatry*, **140**, 1455–1459.
PASNUE & HORTMANN (1983) Psychiatry in Saudi Arabia. *American Journal of Psychiatry*, **140**, 11.
SEBAI, Z. (1985) *Health in Saudi Arabia*. Tihama Publications.
WORLD HEALTH ORGANIZATION (1978) *Mental Disorders: Glossary and Guide to their Classification in Accordance with the Ninth Revision of the International Classification of Diseases* (ICD–9). Geneva: WHO.

10 The Palestinians: under occupation

EYAD EL-SARRAJ

Both the Arabs and the Israelis trace their origins back to their patriarch Abraham. The Hebrew tribes known as the Children of Israel embarked on the conquest of Canaan (as Palestine was then known) in the 13th and 12th centuries BC, at about the same time as the Philistines (from whom the name *Palestine* derives) were taking possession of the coastal area. The Israelite kingdom reached its peak under King David around 1000 BC, before splitting into a northern kingdom and the southern kingdom of Judah. After some centuries of subjection to other powers, an attempt to restore an independent kingdom ended with the Roman conquest of the area in 63 BC. Over a century later, the Romans undertook the reconquest of the country, taking Jerusalem by storm and destroying its temple. After further revolts, the Emperor Hadrian finally expelled all Jews from Jerusalem in AD 135.

The Arab Muslim conquest of Palestine was completed in AD 640, but it took over a century for the majority of the population to embrace the Muslim faith (10–15% of Palestinians still adhere to Christianity). The first four Muslim caliphs (i.e. successors to the prophet Mohammed) ruled from Arabia, after which Damascus became the seat of the Arab Empire. Except for the interlude when a series of crusader kingdoms ruled parts of the eastern Mediterranean basin in the 12th and 13th centuries, the region remained under a succession of Muslim regimes, including for 400 years the Ottoman Turks, until the end of World War I.

The conflict in Palestine in the 20th century has been a struggle between two peoples, the Palestinians and the Jews, for the same piece of land. The Jews, seeking a haven from persecution and discrimination, wanted a state of their own in Palestine, a land that was occupied and ruled by their forefathers. The central problem was that Palestine had been a home for the Palestinians for over a millennium.

In 1947, the United Nations decided on the partition of Palestine. Although the Palestinians rejected partition, and demanded that the matter be referred to the International Court of Justice, the state of Israel was established and the Palestinian refugee problem created. Since the Six Day War of 1967, the Palestinian population of the West Bank and the Gaza Strip has lived under Israeli occupation. There has been much international controversy over the treatment and rights of the Palestinians, particularly over their land and water rights, restrictions on agricultural production, deportations, the right to vote, and the expression of national identity.

In December 1987, the Palestinian uprising (the *Intifada*) began in the occupied West Bank and Gaza. This uprising is a mass movement of civil disobedience and rebellion against the continued occupation, intended to break the economic dependence on Israel by discouraging Palestinian purchase of Israeli products and by developing local or home economies. The Intifada has led to considerable, much publicised conflict with the Israeli authorities. In its first two years, approximately 900 Palestinians were shot and killed, 54% of them children under the age of 14; 22 000 were physically injured and 55 000 detained.

Population changes

On the West Bank, the population increased from 651 800 in 1968 to 934 400 at the end of 1985. Meanwhile, the population in the Gaza Strip increased from 356 800 to 525 500. The average annual growth rate in this period was 2.4% in the West Bank and 3.1% in the Gaza Strip.

Children under the age of 14 constitute 48% of the total population, while the age group 20–34 years forms 23%. This difference is largely due to migration of men, mainly to other Arab states. The fertility rate has not been published, but other rates (child:woman ratio, birth rates) suggest that fertility decreased between 1982 and 1984 by 2% in the West Bank and 4% in Gaza. The ratio of males to females within the age group 40–44 years is very low: 551 males for every 1000 females. Once again, the difference between the two figures represents migration, largely for economic and political reasons.

According to the United Nations Relief and Work Agency's 1986 "Annual Report", the population of registered refugees in the West Bank is 365 315, the majority living in ten refugee camps. In Gaza, the number of refugees is 435 478, living in eight camps.

Indices of health

Infant mortality rate

In Gaza and the West Bank, the infant mortality rate is a subject of controversy, with the Israelis and Palestinians each producing their own figures. Nevertheless, there would be little disagreement with a figure of 65 per 1000 live births.

Nutritional status

In the rural area around Jerusalem, the rate of malnutrition among Palestinians under the age of three has been estimated at 34%. The rate of low birth weight is 20% and anaemia affects 20% of mothers. The majority of malnourished cases are mild to moderate in severity and might easily pass unnoticed by health care providers. According to UNRWA (1986), the rate of underweight children below the age of five in the West Bank and Gaza was 5% (1984 figures).

Parasite infestation

This is a major public health hazard in the occupied areas. According to 1976 Israeli Government figures, the rate of infestation among schoolchildren in Gaza was 50%.

Eye diseases

The rate of binocular blindness is 1.7%, eight times the rate in Great Britain. Single-eye impairment is found at a rate of 6.8%; 28.4% of those examined were infected with trachoma.

Health services

The occupying 'civil administration' includes the Departments of Health, Education, Transport, and Tax which are run by Israeli officers in charge of Palestinian civil servants. Government hospitals are generally understaffed, overcrowded, and short of facilities. During the Intifada, the medical services have been stretched to their limits.

Discrepancies exist in health resources between Israel and the occupied territories. In 1986, the doctor:population ratio for the West Bank and Gaza was 8:10 000, compared with 28:10 000 in Israel. There were more than 200 unemployed Palestinian doctors in the territories. Salaries of Palestinian health workers are low, a doctor's salary being approximately £250 per month, half of it in allowances which do not contribute towards pensions. Expenditure on the health services of Gaza and the West Bank is US$30 per person per year. In Israel itself, salaries are 2–3 times higher and the equivalent expenditure is US$350 (Benevisti, 1986).

The West Bank

In the West Bank, there are nine government hospitals staffed by 132 doctors, 116 nurses, 182 nursing aides, and others. Total beds in 1985 numbered 951. The UNRWA has run a clinic in every refugee camp since the occupation began and has 60 beds allocated in two private hospitals.

The private and national (Palestinian) sector in the West Bank is much more active and expanding. Private clinics and national medical institutions and medical relief committees, supported by foreign governments and agencies, have spread their medical services in the West Bank, especially in the wake of the Intifada. In many cases, however, there is an overlap of services and a lack of co-ordination: some areas have a high concentration of clinics, while others remain deficient.

Gaza Strip

The health services in Gaza are provided by three main groups: the Israeli authorities, the UNRWA, and the private sector. The UNRWA provides free primary health care to the refugees in the eight camps throughout the Strip, along with other services such as primary education, food, and clothing. In every camp, there is an out-patient clinic, usually staffed by one or two doctors and a few nurses; in some of these clinics, there are maternity units. The load of patients in these clinics is overwhelming – up to 150 per day; they also have to take care of vaccinations and the rehydration of children suffering from gastroenteritis. Refugees who need hospital care are referred to the government, or *Ahli*, hospitals.

Every government or UNRWA doctor has the right to operate his or her own private consulting rooms, and everyone does. In reality, doctors pay much more attention to their private patients, a practice that has given the profession a poor reputation.

The *Ahli*-Arab hospital is an ancient hospital that was part of the Baptist Mission in Gaza. It is now the only Palestinian-administered hospital, with a capacity of 75 beds, mainly surgical. With few exceptions, the hospitals of the Gaza Strip were built before 1967. Since the occupation, the absolute increase in the number of beds has been 50, i.e. 6%, and the population increase of 70% has resulted in the bed:population ratio falling to a level of 1.3 per 1000. But if the absolute bed per population ratio appears inadequate, the actual availability of beds to the general population is even worse. Shortly after the occupation, free medical services were abolished and patients requiring hospital admission began to pay bed charges, or have their expenses covered by public health insurance. However, over the years, the insurance premiums and bed charges have risen, the latter to US$170 per night.

The government hospitals in the Gaza Strip are:

Shifa Hospital in Gaza City General Hospital (300 beds)
Children's Hospital (70 beds)

The TB Hospital in Buraij (50% UNRWA – 70 beds)
Nasser Hospital (300 beds)
The Mental Hospital (200 beds)
The Ophthalmic Hospital (25 beds)

In addition, there are 25 clinics throughout the Gaza Strip providing primary health services to holders of government insurance – about 20% of the population. Each clinic is run by a doctor and two or three nurses and nursing aide staff. Some are periodically visited by a paediatrician and a chest specialist. Some have their own pharmacy and laboratory facilities.

Mental health and mental health services

There are no available epidemiological data on the psychiatric morbidity of the Palestinian population. However, those working in the region believe that during the occupation, before the Intifada, stress-related disorders were increasingly reported, depression being the most common, followed by anxiety states. In my clinic alone, we treated approximately 10 000 cases of depression between 1978 and 1985. In addition, drug addiction spread among the young and in the last nine months of 1987, we saw about 300 cases of cocaine addiction.

Another disturbing development was the apparent increase in aggressive, antisocial behaviour which led to families and clans being plagued by infighting. Homicide increased in the Gaza Strip from six cases in 1967 to 66 in 1985. Serious car accidents became common. Suicide, however, continued to be almost non-existent, because of the strong religious belief in the sanctity of life. The social attitude of the Palestinians during this time appeared to grow increasingly fatalistic.

It is also the impression of local health workers that the Intifada has been socially therapeutic: social cohesion has replaced the infighting. Depression and hopelessness have appeared to be replaced by national pride and optimism.

Traditional healers were, in the early years of the occupation, the first line of mental health care. Today, the non-traditional mental health services in the West Bank and Gaza are mainly provided by government health services and a few privately owned psychiatric clinics.

The West Bank

There is only one mental hospital on the West Bank, situated in Bethlehem and containing 320 beds. This represents a figure of 0.04 beds per 1000 population of the West Bank. In 1984, the bed occupancy of Bethlehem Hospital was 120%. The number of patients admitted that year was 880, treated by 7 doctors, 54 nurses and 14 paramedical professionals.

There is a psychiatric out-patient clinic in Bethlehem, another in the Nablus area, and a third in Hebron. There are no community mental health centres as such, no programmes for in-service training or education, and no research work. In Jerusalem, there are three private psychiatric clinics, but no data are available on their activities.

Gaza

Until 1979, psychiatric services in Gaza were mainly assigned to a general practitioner, whose role was to refer psychiatric patients to the West Bank for admission and treatment, while treating mild cases of neurosis and depression locally. In 1979, the Israeli authorities agreed to open a 20-bed in-patient unit by taking over part of the Gaza Eye Hospital. Unfortunately, this unit remained understaffed with one specialist psychiatrist, one junior doctor, eight nurses, three psychologists, and no social workers. There was an out-patient clinic in Gaza and another in Khan Younis in the southern part of the Strip. On admission, patients were looked after mainly by their families; there were permanent shortages of drugs and no ECT apparatus. Local donations were not permitted, nor was help from international agencies.

In 1984, the unit was expanded to 32 beds, and another doctor, five nurses, and two more psychologists were added to the staff. However, the hospital remained overcrowded, with an occupancy rate of 125%, and the average stay of patients was 12 days. Research has been severely limited because of the demand for clinical service.

Conclusion

A mental health programme for the Gaza Strip has been embarked upon. In the initial stages, the target group has been children and the emphasis has been on family interventions. The programme has also included training designed for mental health workers and other involved groups. Additional activities are documentation of progress and research. The Gaza Community Mental Health Project is now seeking collaboration with academic institutions in other parts of the world.

Reference

BENEVISTI, M. (1986) *The West Bank Data Project Report*. Boulder, CO: Westview Press.

11 Egypt: the pace of life and the pace of reform

NASSER LOZA and IMAN NABIL

The Arab Republic of Egypt is one of the largest Middle Eastern countries, with a total area of over one million square kilometres, mostly desert, and less than 4% cultivated land. It is bounded to the north by the Mediterranean, to the south by the Sudan, to the east by the Red Sea and to the west by Libya, and is divided into three geographical zones: the Nile valley, the eastern desert and the western desert. Its long coasts on the Mediterranean and the Red Sea are relatively uninhabited.

Egyptians (1988 population census: 52.9 million) have traditionally lived in the fertile delta and Nile Valley. It is estimated that over 97% of the population lives on 6% of the land and this uneven distribution of the population has resulted in a population density as high as 28 000/km^2 in Cairo, a classic example of high metropolitan primacy. The country is divided into 26 governorates.

Illiteracy was one of the main problems in Egypt until the 1950s, but the education system has expanded rapidly during the past three decades following the introduction of free education at all levels after the 1952 revolution. However, 50% of the present general population still cannot read (Table 11.1).

Egypt has made progress in traditional industries, namely spinning and weaving, as well as in the engineering, metallurgical, chemical, and petroleum industries. Newly discovered oil and gas deposits in Lower Egypt, the western desert and the Red Sea are an important advance for Egyptian

TABLE 11.1
Educational status of the Egyptian population

Educational status	Male: %	Female: %	Total: %
Illiterate	37.8	61.8	49.3
Able to read and write	30.4	18.0	24.4
Qualifications other than degrees	26.0	17.5	21.9
University graduates and above	5.8	2.8	4.4

(Source: Central Agency for Public Mobilisation and Statistics, 1989)

petroleum production. The percentage of total capital investment allocated for the industrial sector amounts to 26% (as opposed to 5% for health services).

Health and health care

The 1952 revolution, which overthrew the government of King Farouk, was a major turning-point in the history of Egypt, as the political system changed from monarchy to republic. The first elected president, Gamal Abdel Nasser, totally restructured the system, introducing one-party rule, an elected parliament, an appointed prime minister, and ministers in all domains. The Ministry of Health has representative offices in every governorate.

However, state-delivered health services are not new in Egypt. Ever since the ancient civilisation of Pharaonic Egypt, successive governments have pledged to improve the quality of their health care. The priests of Pharaonic Egypt took over this role from their temples (Ghalioungy, 1963). Later, in the Islamic era (7th–16th century AD), the state hospitals (*'Bimaristans'*) offered the benefits of modern medicine free of charge to the poor. Of particular fame were their services in the fields of ophthalmology and the care of the insane (Baashar, 1975).

Today the state still assumes the responsibility of ensuring quality health services for all citizens. But with only 3% of the population over 65 years (Table 11.2), and a birth rate of 37.5 per 1000, health services have placed priority on child care and birth control.

TABLE 11.2
Age structure of the Egyptian population

Age in years	Percentage of population
Less than 6	19
6–12	15
12–65	63
65 and over	3

(Source: Central Agency for Public Mobilisation and Statistics, 1989)

To meet this responsibility, the following policies have been adopted:

(a) The extension of health services to the rural areas
(b) Special programmes to combat endemic diseases, particularly bilharziasis and tuberculosis
(c) The extension of free health services in rural and urban areas
(d) Children's and mothers' welfare centres

(e) Medical services to all citizens in state hospitals at nominal fees and a significant increase in the number of beds in these hospitals.

These policies, however, have done little to improve the quality of care in state hospitals and any improvement in health services is rapidly overtaken as a result of the population increase (Table 11.3).

TABLE 11.3
Population statistics and hospital provision since 1952

	1952	1983	1984	1985	1986	1987	1988
Number of hospital beds	35 744	90 445	92 003	92 700	94 354	98 344	100 406
Population estimate: thousands	21 437	45 721	46 990	48 349	49 863	51 297	52 919
Birth rate per thousand population	45.2	36.8	38.6	39.8	38.7	37.9	37.5
Death rate per thousand population	17.8	9.7	9.5	9.4	9.2	8.6	8.6
Natural population increase	27.4	27.1	29.1	30.4	29.5	29.3	28.9

(Source: Central Agency for Public Mobilisation and Statistics, 1989)

Mental health

Psychiatric services in Egypt are poorly funded and understaffed, with only one psychiatrist for every 300 000 citizens and one psychiatric bed for every 7000 individuals (Okasha, 1989).

The load on these facilities has been increased in recent years by the rising problem of drug abuse in Egypt. Since the early 1980s, heroin has been affecting mostly young men. The work of helping drug addicts in Egypt is carried out primarily by psychiatrists. The problem is seen as essentially medical and the role of social and community workers is limited.

Services are delivered through three main systems, which are outlined below.

The ministry of health hospitals

These offer many services in large overcrowded hospitals in Cairo and Alexandria, and in smaller psychiatric departments, which often consist of out-patient clinics in general hospitals in the governorates. Services are offered free or for nominal fees, but shortage of staff and medication, as well as limited facilities, all contribute to making any attempt at improvement a difficult task.

The university teaching hospitals

There are eight university departments of psychiatry, each with associated teaching hospitals, and these have the dual role of training and licensing psychiatric practitioners.

They offer a diploma in psychiatry as well as a Master of Sciences (MSc) and a Medical Doctorate (MD). The teaching hospitals offer little in-patient care; some have no beds at all and others have no more than a handful of beds for male patients only.

Private clinics

Private practice in psychiatry is extensive: almost all qualified psychiatrists, including university staff and professors, are at least partly involved in private work. The service is offered mainly through private consulting rooms in most cities. There are several private hospitals in Cairo offering good standards of care with multidisciplinary teams working under consultants, many of whom received their psychiatric training abroad. Unfortunately, this quality of care is available only to a small minority of the population.

Use of psychiatric services

Patients can present themselves, without referral, to any private or state – Ministry of Health or university – clinic. Although figures on the percentage of the population using each service are not available, by a rough estimate less than 10% of the population have access to a private psychiatric practice. Patients requiring out-patient services can obtain adequate care in both private and state hospitals. For patients needing hospital admission, however, the situation is different. The average Egyptian household cannot afford private in-patient care, so patients are likely to present to the large state mental hospitals in Cairo. These huge institutions, providing an insufficient number of beds to cover the needs of the whole country, have been the subject of major controversy.

The government has plans to close the two largest psychiatric hospitals in the country (the Abasseya and the Khanka hospitals), but the psychiatrists' associations are concerned about the lack of funding for adequate community care. Although they believe that the present provision is inadequate, admission to large institutions is considered better than having psychiatric patients in the community with no support (Loza & Nabil, 1990).

Plans for psychiatric services in Egypt in the year 2000 must address this issue, and the closure of the large mental hospitals should only be contemplated if and when adequate alternative services have been established in the community. A good compromise would be to improve the conditions of state psychiatric hospitals, possibly by first setting up smaller hospitals in the governorates and then closing the large hospitals in Cairo.

Planning for the future

One of the main problems facing Egypt is the rapid increase in population which impedes development efforts and frustrates the hopes of improving the quality of life of every Egyptian. Any plan aimed at improving health care will have to make a priority of birth control. The Supreme Council for Family Planning was established in 1965 to coordinate activities with the Family Planning Board and its 37 509 health units located throughout the country in making family-planning methods available at nominal prices. Yet traditional religious concepts still prevail, and population increase is a long way from being controlled. Education and communication programmes have an important role to play in this field.

Specifically, plans aiming to improve psychiatric services in Egypt need to consider three aspects:

(a) Psychiatric education and training
(b) Services for addiction
(c) Clinical services to the patient, both in hospitals, and in the community.

Psychiatric education

The training of Egyptian doctors in psychiatry is not new; the MSc degree in psychiatry and neurology has been offered by Cairo University for most of this century. Egypt has traditionally supplied neighbouring Middle-Eastern countries with qualified psychiatrists to run their services. Medical and psychiatric education in Egypt is in English. As the name of the degree implies, neurology and psychiatry are not taught as separate disciplines, but in practice students tend to choose their own area of interest. In the MD degree the two disciplines are separated.

Plans to improve psychiatric education in Egypt would need to change little of the academic content of existing programmes. Egyptian textbooks in psychiatry include the most up-to-date basic knowledge, although there are minor deficiencies in some subspecialties.

A step forward would be to 'decentralise' the training institutions. Currently, only the university departments are officially recognised. These departments, although undoubtedly staffed by tutors with good teaching skills, lack basic facilities for clinical training, such as enough hospital beds and good nursing standards; some have no in-patient facilities. Ideally, these university tutors should take their talents into the overcrowded state hospitals where both patients and students could benefit from their skills. This would gradually improve training as well as patient care in these centres.

Another advantage of such a step would be a change from the current practice whereby a candidate is both trained and examined by the same tutors in his own centre, a situation that raises questions of impartiality in the examinations.

Addiction

Addiction is rapidly affecting Egyptian society, and consequently psychiatric practice. Young people are the main persons affected, and heroin is the most popular and dangerous drug used. The long coasts of Egypt facilitate smuggling of drugs, particularly following the loosening of border controls after the end of the war with Israel.

The government has realised the short-term and long-term impact of the problem in its medical, economic and psychological aspects. Strict laws, enforced by capital punishment for drug trafficking, have been applied. Help for drug addicts is delivered in the districts as part of their psychiatric services, but poor funding and lack of experienced personnel make the quality of care inadequate. An improvement in the management of drug addicts in Egypt will have to include a more significant use of social workers as well as the introduction of self-help groups.

Clinical services

No national psychiatric service scheme can depend entirely on private practice. There is an urgent need for an improvement in the current condition of state psychiatric hospitals. Recently, the media have exposed the problem, with the result that there is much controversy regarding the ideal solution. Politicians have supported community psychiatry, arguing for the benefits of caring for the mentally ill in the community rather than admitting them to hospital. As in the West, psychiatrists contend that this may be the government's economic solution to the problem, but that this could allow a denial of its responsibility for patients' welfare.

Community psychiatry is of course a good solution only when enough money is spent on it. Community psychiatric services should include everything from doctors and nurses to sending meals to patients at home. Community services should be developed primarily around a family-orientated support scheme, with community psychiatric personnel available to visit families and offer basic help in the form of medication and simple psychotherapeutic advice. In Egypt, it would be unwise not to make good use of family and community support for the chronically ill, since Egyptian families have always accommodated their psychiatrically ill members. The slow, regular pace of life of the Egyptian *fellah* (peasant) in the Nile Valley is often a haven for psychiatric patients.

References

BAASHAR, T. (1975) The Arab countries. In *World History of Psychiatry* (ed. T. G. Howells). New York, London: Churchill Livingstone.

CENTRAL AGENCY FOR PUBLIC MOBILISATION AND STATISTICS (1989) *Statistical Yearbook for 1989*. Cairo, Egypt: Central Agency for Public Mobilisation and Statistics.

GHALIOUNGY, P. (1963) *Magic and Medical Science in Ancient Egypt*. London: Hodder and Stoughton.

LOZA, N. & NABIL, I. (1990) Psychiatric services in Egypt: scope for improvement. *Business Monthly*, **6** (no. 4), 17–18.

OKASHA, A. (1989) The role of psychiatry in mental health policy formulation. An Egyptian perspective. In *Psychiatry Today. Accomplishments and Promises. VIII World Congress of Psychiatry, Athens 1989*, p. 1791. Excerpta Medica International Congress Series. Amsterdam: Elsevier.

12 Libya: a challenge ahead

FAREJ M. MAHDAWI and ALI M. EL ROEY

Libya is located in North Africa in an area of 1 762 000 km², with 1900 km of Mediterranean coast. The southern mountains and deserts occupy two-thirds of the country, the other third being the fertile agricultural plains of the north. Its climate is as varied as its geography, from a warm and rainy (in winter) north to a hot and arid south.

The population of Libya in 1990 was 4 080 000 (*Encyclopaedia Britannica*), 75% of whom live in the main northern cities of the country (Tripoli, Benghazi, and Musrata). The population growth is 3.45% annually. Further sociodemographic information can be found in Table 12.1. The Libyan people are part of the Arabic nation and the social structure is based on extended families and tribes. All Libyans originate from old Arab tribes; the official religion is Islam and the language is Arabic.

TABLE 12.1
Sociodemographic features of Libya

	Percentage of population
Sex distribution	
male	51.04
female	48.98
Age distribution	
below 15 years	51.4
15 years to 34 years	25.5
35 years to 54 years	15.3
55 years to 64 years	3.6
Above 65 years	4.2
Marital status (population aged over 15 years)	
Single	21.6
Married	69.4
Divorced	2.6
Widowed	6.3

(Source: Population data, 1984 census)

Education is free in Libya. Basic education (six primary years and three preparatory years) is compulsory for all Libyans above six years of age. Secondary school education (three years) is provided through general, technical, agricultural, management and financial schools. Higher education is dispensed by many colleges and seven universities. There are 23 000 university students (Al Arab, 1989). The total number of students in Libya in 1986 was 1 293 000, about 32% of the total population.

The Libyans celebrate various social and religious events such as marriage, childbirth, going to Mecca for hajj, Ramadan nights, and *Eid* days (holidays following the fasting month of Ramadan in Muslim religion). There are two television channels, in English and French respectively, in addition to the main Arabic channel.

The Libyan economy depends mainly on oil exports and petrochemical industrial products. The GNP (gross national product) was approximately US$22 326 million in 1987 (*Encyclopaedia Britannica*). The income per capita was US$5500 in 1987. Although the main source of income is petrol, most Libyans work in agriculture (olives, palm and citrus trees, and cereals) in the coastal strip as well as in other parts of the country.

The history of Libya follows the history of all mankind, as many of the ancient civilisations passed through the country. Among the old civilisations known to have flourished in Libya are the Jarmanite in the south and the Libo and the Maccay in the north. A number of invaders have attacked Libya over the centuries. The Greeks built the famous five eastern cities, some of them still open to tourists (e.g. Cyrine), and the Phoenicians invaded the west, where they built the three cities of Sebrata, Oia (Tripoli) and Leptus Magna. Later, the Romans conquered the whole country and stayed until the Islamic conquest, which connected Libyan and Islamic history. In the early 15th century, the Ottomans extended their empire, which thereafter included Libya for more than four centuries, until 1911 when Italy invaded, although resistance from the people of Libya continued for over 25 years.

In 1936 Omar El Mukhtar, the 70-year-old leader of Libyan resistance, was hanged in public, an event witnessed by many people at Benghazi (Salugue). During World War II, Libya became a battlefield, Tobruk being just one of the many battle sites. When the war ended, the country was under the Allied forces' administration until the UN recognised its independence in 1951. Libya was then ruled by a King from the Sanussi Royal Family until, following the revolution of 1 September 1969, it became a republic. In 1977, it became the Socialist People's Libyan Arab Jamahiriya.

Libyan culture does not differ from that of any other Arabic and Islamic society in its norms, beliefs and attitudes. Parents are at the head of the family and elder brothers are their substitutes. The role of women has changed from that of mother and housewife to one of partnership in many aspects of life, including employment in positions of responsibility in society. Marriages are usually arranged by families – a practice associated with marital problems which affect children and society as a whole. The extended family plays an important role in providing long-term support to relatives who need it, such as the chronically ill or bereaved. Religion also offers support to believers in coping with daily life. According to Islamic religion, suicide is a major sin, and alcohol or indeed any substance which makes the person lose control of him/herself is prohibited. Homosexuality is also prohibited.

Health and health services

All public services are free but there are also private clinics which are run on a fee-for-service basis. Public services are financed by the State, and the total budget for the health service varies from one year to another according to specific needs or projects. In 1980 the health expenditure per person per year was US $120.00 (Department of Planning, Secretariat of Health, 1981).

The structure of the health services is similar to that found in Western countries. There are specialised hospitals, general hospitals in the main cities (200–500 beds), district hospitals in small towns (100–200 beds), and health clinics in the main cities and towns. The total number of beds was 22 007 beds (6.8 beds per 1000 population) in 1980 (Department of Planning, Secretariat of Health, 1981).

Medical education is delivered by medical universities, such as the Al Arab Medical University at Benghazi, and two medical schools that are part of larger universities (Al Fateh and Sebha). There are 1200 medical students, and all medical and scientific teaching is in English. A medical degree of MBBS is obtained after passing the final examinations supervised by experts brought from the UK and other countries. The curriculum includes one year of pre-medical study, five years of full-time academic study plus clinical teaching, and a one-year internship at an approved teaching hospital. There are 4987 doctors, i.e. one per 710 population (Al Arab, 1989), 12 770 nurses and 1791 technicians and assistant nurses (Department of Planning, Secretariat of Health, 1981).

The infant mortality rate was 37 per 1000 in 1979. The leading causes of death in adults were cerebrovascular accidents, road traffic accidents, other cardiovascular diseases, and malignancies (Department of Planning, Secretariat of Health, 1981).

Mental health services

Mental health services in Libya are delivered mainly through the two leading psychiatric hospitals in the country (Benghazi and Tripoli), and through psychiatric units at general hospitals. A national committee for mental health was recently appointed, and it is hoped it will have an important role in the promotion and planning of mental health services and activities throughout the country. There is no mental health act in Libya, although the National Committee for Mental Health is currently preparing a workshop to discuss the need for one. The principles of general law are applied to psychiatric patients.

The two main psychiatric hospitals, both of which are teaching centres affiliated to universities, are:

(a) *Tripoli (Ave Sina) Hospital,* located in the city, with 1200 beds and out-patient facilities run within the hospital. It caters for the south-western part of the country

(b) *Benghazi Hospital* is a 350-bed extension of the old Gawarsha hospital which now accommodates the chronic patients. It was built beside other teaching hospitals and the Al-Arab Medical University buildings 12 km from the city centre. It has an emergency service open 24 hours a day and four clinical teams with their own record-keeping and out-patient departments available at health clinics in the city.

In addition, there is a 40-bed psychiatric unit at Sebha General Hospital and 20-bed psychiatric units in the cities of El Marj, Derna, Misurata and Zwaia. The total number of psychiatric beds in Libya is 1670. Rehabilitation and occupational therapy units will be set up in psychiatric hospitals and other centres in the near future.

Mental health services suffer from a huge manpower shortage but there are no official figures. Benghazi Hospital had four consultants (two Libyans), 14 junior doctors (eight Libyans), 80 nurses (two Libyans), 10 psychologists (all Libyans) and one social worker in 1985 (El Roey & Mahdawi, 1985).

Benghazi Psychiatric Hospital organises and runs training programmes, among them a one-month programme for fourth-year medical students and other courses for postgraduate psychology and social services students. Postgraduate teaching for junior psychiatric doctors is given at Benghazi Hospital in the form of lectures and case conferences. The psychiatric unit of Al-Arab Medical University, in conjunction with Benghazi Hospital's Training and Education Unit, has presented a short introductory course for primary health care doctors annually since 1985.

A psychiatric nursing school began teaching 25 students in 1990. Teaching is provided by qualified psychologists and psychiatrists, members of the university staff supported by visiting professors from the United Kingdom, India and Egypt.

Research is scarce. A unique study carried out by a team of researchers from Benghazi Psychiatric Hospital examined 100 consecutive cases of hysteria, the great majority under 21 years of age and presenting with pseudoseizures. The authors concluded that hysterical symptoms in Libya should be viewed as a form of illness behaviour which is more culturally acceptable than psychological complaints as a reason for consultation (El Roey *et al*, 1986).

Libyan culture has made its own contributions to the treatment of mentally ill people. Amulets which contain verses of the Holy Koran, and the reading of parts of the Koran, are traditionally prescribed for neurotic and reactive psychological problems. The traditional healers in Libya still have a role in mental health through their non-religious methods of treatment (spiritual or magic). Visiting a shrine to dead sheiks is, for example, a treatment used by people who have a mental or physical illness. The pilgrimage to the Sacred House, Mecca, is believed to relieve all past sins and wrongful acts.

Most mentally ill people present to doctors in clinics or hospitals with somatic symptoms such as headaches or breathlessness, rather than mood disturbance (El Islam, 1984). The stigma of being mentally ill, a universal problem, prevents many treatable patients from approaching psychiatric services during the early stages of their illnesses. Many patients seek help only when their social performance has deteriorated so much that it cannot be hidden any more.

Few epidemiological data are available, but hospital records at Benghazi Hospital can give an estimate of the most common causes of admission (see Table 12.2). The majority of the patients admitted are males (69%) from urban settings (84%).

TABLE 12.2
Diagnoses of patients presenting to Benghazi Psychiatric Hospital (1985)

Diagnosis	Percentage of admissions
Schizophrenic psychosis	38.75
Affective psychosis	16.85
Neurotic disorders	11.50
Acute psychoses	8.62
Organic psychotic conditions	7.33
Mental retardation	5.05
Paranoid states	3.27
Personality disorders	3.07
Drug dependence	1.19
Others	4.36

Conclusion

The National Programme of Mental Health (El Roey & Ahmedoni, 1985) has summarised the priorities, targets and plan of action, and given a broad and comprehensive view on mental health in Libya. The main problems are shortage of staff and lack of facilities, social stigma and centralisation of services. These problems could be greatly improved through the enhancement of the primary care network.

Since the main problem seems to be manpower shortage, a special effort should be undertaken to train more health personnel and community members such as teachers to deliver psychiatric services. The national programme has addressed these problems and given detailed information and guidelines on how to overcome the manpower problem. International agencies and developed countries are crucial in providing advice and cooperation with local training initiatives for all types of health workers. The World Health Organization has also started to provide advice on mental health services.

Acknowledgements

I wrote this paper while on a WHO fellowship. I would like to express my special thanks to the WHO Mental Health Offices in Libya, Alexandria and Geneva. I would also like to thank all my colleagues at Benghazi Psychiatric Hospital.

References

AL ARAB MAGAZINE (1989) *Special Issue on Libya*. London: Al Arab Publications.
DEPARTMENT OF PLANNING, SECRETARIAT OF HEALTH (1981) *Health for all People*. Tripoli, Libya: The Arabic Book Establishment.
EL ISLAM, M. F. (1984) Some transcultural aspects of depression in Arabic patients. *The Islamic World Medical Journal*, (March), 48–49.
EL ROEY, A. & MAHDAWI, F. (1985) *The Training and Educational Unit*. Benghazi, Libya: Review Books, General Publications and Press Establishment.
——, TINNYUNT PU, M. & MOHAMMED, E. (1986) 100 cases of hysteria in Eastern Libya. *British Journal of Psychiatry*, **148**, 606–609.
—— & AHMEDUNI, M. (1989) *The National Programme of Mental Health for Libya*. Benghazi, Libya: General Publications and Press Establishment.

V. South and Central America

13 Brazil: a giant wakes up to progress and inequality

EDUARDO IACOPONI, RONALDO RAMOS LARANJEIRA and JAIR DE JESUS MARI

Euclides da Cunha, in what has been described as the greatest of Brazilian classics, *"Os Sertões"* (*Revolt in the Backlands*; 1947), wrote:

> "We are condemned to civilization.
> Either we progress or we disappear."

Since the first publication of da Cunha's book in 1902, 13 years after the proclamation of the republic, Brazil has seen a transformation from a quasi-colonial agricultural economy into a modern industrial state, although these two conditions are still seen in parallel in many parts of the country (Leighton, 1986).

Covering an area of approximately 8.5 million km², Brazil occupies 47% of South America and is the fifth largest country in the world. As it has neither inaccessible mountains nor frozen wastes, there is an enormous potential for land use, although over 30% of the country lies in the basin of the river Amazon, with its dense tropical forest in the north of the country. The Amazon area has, until recently, remained virtually unexplored, but in the past decade this region has undergone deforestation, and ecologically damaging industrialisation similar to that observed in Europe and North America in the past two centuries. Fig. 13.1 shows a map of Brazil giving the populations (in millions) of the seven biggest metropolitan areas.

A nation of gigantic contrasts, Brazil today has the eighth largest economy in the West. It is a complex economy which includes the export not only of agricultural goods like coffee and sugar cane, but also of various minerals and manufactured goods, like cars and small aircraft (CACEX, 1988). This economic growth has been partly aided by extensive financial backing from abroad, a trend that has been observed since 1824, only two years after independence from the Portuguese Empire, when the then Brazilian monarchy borrowed £1 million from Britain (Sodré, 1987). Today Brazil has a debt greater than that of any other country in the less developed world.

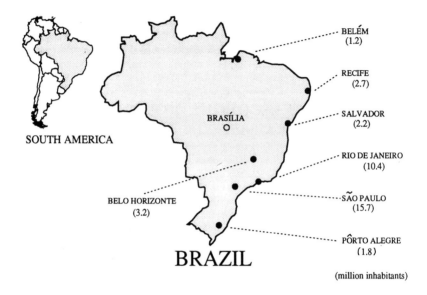

Fig. 13.1. Brazil and its metropolitan areas

In a review published in *The Economist* (Harvey, 1987), the forecast was that the country would soon be the next member of the club of developed nations, an overly optimistic view when other social aspects of the country are considered. Brazil has one of the highest concentrations of wealth: the richer 20% possess 67% of the national income, while the poorer 40% contribute only 7% to the total income (Abranches, 1985). In Greater São Paulo, Brazil's richest industrial and cultural centre, 50% of the population earned less than £240 per month in 1980, and half of these were earning less than £140 per month. In the same year, 500 000 people were living in 680 *favelas* (shanty towns) in the outskirts of the urban area, and another 2 million were living in *cortiços* (the old deteriorating city centre tenements). People living in this sort of accommodation, the urban poor, are inevitably at the bottom end of the range of salaries (SEADE, 1988).

It would be tempting to attribute such levels of poverty and unequal distribution of wealth to the period of military dictatorship that was imposed on the country from 1964 to 1985. Although the wealth of the nation became even more concentrated in the richest sector during the dictatorship years, the unequal pattern of distribution was already profound before the military took power. In fact, this pattern has not changed since the end of the last military presidency and commencement of a new democratic era: wealth has become even more concentrated in the hands of the better off in the recent democratic period from 1985 to 1989, suggesting that the causes of such distribution of wealth are not solely related to the lack of democracy. This immense gap separating the poorest parts of Brazilian society from access to basic human needs is not a recent feature of the nation's history; it goes back to the colonial past and the authoritarian tradition associated with the influence and interests of the colonial empires and the Catholic Church in the New World (Sodré, 1987).

In 1986, Brazil was the sixth most populous nation on earth, with about 136 million inhabitants, 65% of whom were under 30, with a constant migration from rural to urban areas (Durhan, 1978; IBGE, 1988). In the last decade, however, the growth rate of the population has slowly but steadily fallen (Martine, 1989).

Although Brazil has a reputation for being a 'melting pot' with a high degree of social tolerance and social mix, there is still clear evidence of different racial types (Seyferth, 1986), as seen in the 1950 national census, the last to seek racial origins: 61% were white, mainly of European ancestry; 11% were black, descendants of African slaves, and 27% were mulatto, i.e. a mixture of black and white. The remaining 1% were made up from offspring of Japanese, Korean and Taiwanese migrants, with Brazilian Indians accounting for less than 0.2% of the total population.

The blacks and mulattos are over-represented in the underprivileged portion of the society (60%), earning less than twice the national minimum wage – which averages £30 per month. This suggests that, unlike other immigrants, they have not managed to succeed in Brazilian society. None the less, these peoples have had an outstanding impact on many aspects of Brazilian cultural life including music, sports, food, literature and religion (Degler, 1971).

Primary education in Brazil is free and theoretically compulsory, but only one in seven children completes elementary school; one of the reasons for this high drop-out rate is the need to earn money very early in life. Rates of illiteracy vary in the 23 states of the country, but are generally below 25% (for those aged 15 years and over).

Similar variation is observed in the rates of infant mortality: 140 per thousand in the north-eastern rural areas of the country, and 54 per thousand in the more urbanised south (IBGE, 1988). These rates of infant mortality point to one of the major causes of death in the country, malnutrition. In the more developed parts of the country, malnutrition affects 30% of the infant population, while rates of about 70–80% are seen in the less developed north and north-east. In these undernourished children, death occurs after episodes of measles or acute infectious gastroenterocolitis followed by dehydration. Pulmonary tuberculosis is also widespread in Brazil, again affecting mainly the less developed areas in the north, where about 17% (compared with 8% in the south) of the population is infected, although fewer develop the full symptoms of the disease. Brazil is also severely affected by the tropical diseases like malaria, schistosomiasis and Chagas' disease (trypanosomiasis), three of the major causes of death and disability in the northern part of the country. As has been said before, in some aspects

Brazil has the worst of the two worlds: in the big industrial conurbations the main causes of death are not only those mentioned above, but also those related to sedentary lifestyles (myocardial infarction, cerebrovascular accident), smoking, traffic accidents, and urban violence.

Psychiatric disorders are not the main problems affecting the health of Brazilians. In the following sections, a brief description of the organisation of the health services and the steps necessary to become a psychiatrist in Brazil will be presented, followed by the distribution of psychiatric disorders in various levels of the community and the psychiatric services available at each level.

Health services in Brazil

The formal organisation of state health services in Brazil followed a path which closely resembled that of the more industrialised part of the world. Medical and hospital care, until the beginning of this century, were almost exclusively provided by charities and other voluntary institutions (Luz, 1982). Only after the appearance of Social Security schemes did government participation show a significant increase. Initially, in the 1920s, the railway workmen, and later the Seamen's Pension Fund, were established. This trend then spread to other professional categories and finally, in 1966, all Social Security institutes were amalgamated to form the *Instituto Nacional de Previdência Social* (INPS), which became nationally responsible for the health services for workers (Donnangelo, 1975; Luz, 1978).

Under the INPS, which was dependent on a contribution from employers as well as employees, the administration of the social security and health services became centralised, while the tasks of public health and environmental control were dealt with by the Ministry of Health (Bastos, 1971; Mello, 1977). This Ministry was also responsible for the provision of medical services to the unemployed, the underemployed, and their families (Roemer, 1968, 1986).

Later developments have seen the separation of the health services and social security functions of the INPS (giving birth to the present INAMPS – *Instituto Nacional de Assistência Médica da Previdência Social*) and also the decentralisation of the health services to state and municipal control. For instance, the administration of primary health care services, previously run by the Ministry of Health, was passed over to municipal branches. This is particularly important in understanding the network of primary health care in urban areas like São Paulo, to be described shortly.

There is a substantial participation by the private sector in the delivery of health services in Brazil. Instead of building its own hospitals and out-patient clinics, or directly employing health workers, the INAMPS opted to 'buy' services from the private sector (Cordeiro, 1980). In 1970, only a few years after its creation, the INPS (later to become INAMPS) owned 25 hospitals, but bought services from another 2634 private hospitals. The private sector also runs hospitals and other medical services independently, but these reach only a very small proportion of the population (Iutaka, 1966).

The delivery of health care to different parts of the population in Brazil can be summarised as follows. The richer segment generally uses the private sector and sometimes the services provided by the INAMPS, which also delivers services for the employed segment of the population and their families. The unemployed, the newcomers to the big cities, and others at the poorest end of community, receive care, whenever possible, from state and municipal health services. Organised primary health care in Brazil is an example of government efforts to assist the urban poor.

Doctors and medical education in Brazil

One of the first acts of the King of Portugal, D. João VI, when he arrived in Brazil in 1808, fleeing from the Napoleonic war in Europe, was to create the first Faculty of Medicine, in the state of Bahia. Only seven months later, D. João VI also founded the School of Anatomy, Surgery and Medicine of the Royal Army Hospital, this time in Rio de Janeiro (Salles, 1971).

Following these early foundations, the number of medical schools grew very slowly, and in 1960 there was a total of only 28 schools for the whole country, 15 of them created in the 1950s. The period from 1961 to 1980, however, saw a three fold increase in the number of medical schools (to a total of 75), from which about 9000 new doctors were being produced per year (Fraga-Filho & Rosa, 1980).

In both the medical school curriculum and the training of specialists, the emphasis is on the scientific approach to diseases. Doctors are expected to be technically competent to diagnose and treat diseases in individual patients, *according to international standards* (Landmann, 1983). The majority of textbooks available to medical students, particularly those sponsored by the World Health Organization, are translations from American and European 'classics'. The choice of textbooks for trainees in the medical specialties is more modest, and here the ability to read texts in English is unofficially compulsory.

Medicine is prestigious in Brazil. Every year there are about 100 applicants for each place and the entrance examination involves at the very minimum a good knowledge of biology, physics, and chemistry. Upper-middle-class applicants who have been privately educated are usually more successful, leading to a predominance of white male students, very much as in the more developed countries. It takes at least six years to be medically qualified, and another two to five to specialise (e.g., two years for psychiatry, five years for neurosurgery).

Distribution of doctors in the country

This growth in the number of medical schools was not uniform throughout the country, most of them being located in the richer south-eastern regions like São Paulo and Rio de Janeiro. Doctors graduating from these schools also tended to concentrate their practices in the state capitals or the more urbanised regions of the country (Landmann, 1982). Table 13.1 shows the number of medical schools and doctors in three different regions of Brazil.

It can be seen that the regional differences are immense and even the apparently acceptable number of doctors in the south-eastern region is in fact highly concentrated in the major cities.

TABLE 13.1
Number of medical schools and doctors in three regions of Brazil (in 1979)

	South	South-east	North
No. of medical schools	14	42	3
No. of doctors	11 835	51 046	2123
Proportion of doctors in the capitals	46%	60%	85%
Ratio of doctors:population	1:1843	1:984	1:2248

(Adapted from Landmann, 1982)

Medical specialisation

Due to the pressures for better jobs, particularly in the private sector, there is a strong tendency towards specialisation in Brazil (Sayeg, 1978). This also leads to a concentration of doctors in the urban areas where the better-equipped hospitals and out-patient services are to be found (Banta, 1986). Table 13.2 shows the areas of specialisation that are favoured by doctors in two states of Brazil.

TABLE 13.2
Distribution of the medical specialties in the States of São Paulo and Rio de Janeiro

Specialty	São Paulo (Bussab, 1984) %	Rio de Janeiro (Sayeg, 1978) %
Internal medicine	38.5	16.5
Paediatrics	14.9	9.3
Gynaecology and obstetrics	9.9	15.5
Cardiology	5.0	5.6
Orthopaedic surgery	3.8	0.9
Ophthalmology	3.7	1.2
General surgery	3.6	6.1
Psychiatry	3.3	4.8
Neurology	1.6	0.6
Urology	1.5	0.3
Gastroenterology	1.4	2.5
Endocrinology	0.5	1.7
All others	12.3	35.0
Total number of doctors	25 753	691

Whether the observed differences in the choice of specialty are a consequence of the dissimilar samples of the two studies, or whether they represent the influences of market and other forces, cannot be ascertained from the data in this table.

Specialisation in psychiatry

It is estimated that, on average, 3% of doctors in Brazil specialise in psychiatry, although this rate may be considerably lower in the more rural areas (Bussab, 1984). The total number of psychiatrists in the country is estimated to be around 6000 (Langenbach & Negreiros, 1988).

There are several academic and non-academic services that offer places for junior doctors to specialise in psychiatry. All these places must meet the criteria established by the Ministry of Education, in order to be recognised as training centres. The curriculum for specialisation in psychiatry, prepared by the Ministry of Education, is broadly based on the US model of 'residency', and consists of a minimum of two and a maximum of three years of training, with compulsory rotations in psychiatric hospitals, out-patient units, and emergency units, and strongly recommended shorter rotations in liaison and child psychiatry, neurology, and community and social psychiatry, although not all training centres follow these latter recommendations. The orientation of most centres is towards a more biological approach to the diagnosis and treatment of major psychiatric disorders, although other approaches such as psychodynamic or existentialist psychiatry are also taught.

Doctors interested in practising psychiatry can sit professional examinations organised at a national level by the Brazilian Association of Psychiatrists. However, these are not yet compulsory, and it is still quite common to find doctors working in psychiatric hospitals and private psychiatric clinics who either specialised in other fields of medicine, or have not undergone any formal specialisation. The ready availability of courses in the various branches of psychotherapy, particularly in the big cities, certainly contributes to the phenomenon of non-specialised doctors working as psychiatrists.

Psychiatric services in Brazil

Since the construction in 1852 of the first institution for the mentally ill, with 350 beds, on the outskirts of Rio de Janeiro, the organisation of psychiatric services in Brazil has been almost exclusively orientated towards the psychiatric hospital (Mari, 1983; Resende, 1987), with the last hundred years having seen the building of dozens of macro hospitals in various regions of Brazil, usually located just outside growing urban areas.

Recently, however, there have been several government initiatives to substantially alter this picture. Attempts to enhance the currently small contribution of community services and the primary care system have been set in action as well as the creation of psychiatric units in general hospitals (DINSAM, 1987). Improvements in community psychiatry are already evident in some parts of Brazil, but the situation is still far from reaching the whole nation.

To aid the description of psychiatric services in Brazil, two strategies will be followed. Firstly, the model proposed by Goldberg & Huxley (1980) which describes the possible pathways of psychiatric care at various levels in the community will be adopted (Fig. 13.2). Secondly, instead of describing how these levels of care occur throughout the country, a few specific examples of psychiatric services in different regions of Brazil will be given. Generalisations of psychiatric services in the country as a whole therefore cannot be made from these examples.

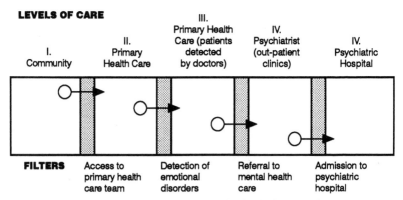

Fig. 13.2. Goldberg and Huxley's model of psychiatric disorders in the community

Level I – Psychiatry in the community

Epidemiological estimates

The understanding of the impact and distribution of psychiatric disorders in a community begins with the measure of the prevalence and incidence rates obtained from epidemiological surveys. In the north-east of the country, Santana (1982) used standardised instruments to study the prevalence of psychiatric disorders in a suburb of Salvador, the sixth largest metropolitan region in Brazil, with 2.2 million inhabitants. The overall prevalence rate for adults was 20.2%, with women and migrants being more at risk than other subgroups. In the southern state of Rio Grande do Sul, a prevalence rate of 25% was obtained for the neuroses, while schizophrenia and major depression, both under DSM–III diagnoses (American Psychiatric Association, 1980), accounted for 0.6% and 0.8%, respectively, of the total adult population living in the state (SSMA/RS, 1989). Other community studies conducted in various parts of Brazil have been reviewed by Almeida-Filho *et al* (1988), and the rates of prevalence of psychiatric disorders usually remained around the 20% level.

Drinking problems and alcoholism have also been subjected to community surveys; in Salvador (Santana, 1982), 14.2% of the interviewed sample of adults were making daily use of alcohol, while 9.7% were described as displaying drunken behaviour at least once a week. The rates of prevalence of alcoholism and drinking problems in other parts of the country varied wildly, and it has been suggested that this variation is more a consequence of dissimilar methods employed by investigators than of true differences in morbidity (Santana & Almeida-Filho, 1987).

Alternative approaches to medicine and popular medicine

The first level of psychiatric care accessible to the community in Brazil, particularly to the urban poor, is, almost without exception, the non-official network of popular and spiritual medicine (Argandoña & Kiev, 1972; Ngokwey, 1988). The middle and upper classes have access to various options of official and alternative medicine, all privately delivered. Among the alternative options, homeopathy, anthroposophy and acupuncture are the most fashionable.

On the other hand, the urban poor tend to use a different path of non-official health care. When in physical and mental distress, they sometimes try to find cures for ailments at:

(a) the centres of African religions (like *umbanda* and *candomblé* – see Montero, 1985)
(b) the *benzedeiras*, local spiritual healers who also make use of curative herbs
(c) the pharmacist in a local chemist's shop.

Brandão (1984) has suggested that, for the urban poor, the selection of provider varies according to the type of ailment: problems recognised as being more physical and acute, like fractures of the bones and appendicitis, are treated by the doctors in official medicine; problems like mental disturbances, nervousness, and abdominal pain are in the domain of the religious healer; and minor symptoms and disorders such as headache, common cold, and gastroenteritis are taken to the pharmacist. However, other studies have shown that there is not such a well defined preference of health care, or a hierarchical sequence chosen by the patients: rather, they often ask for advice from all available sources, including the doctors of the official health services.

Level II – Psychiatry in primary health care

Epidemiological estimates

Very seldom has the topic of psychiatry and primary care in Brazil been submitted to a methodological approach. It was only recently that psychiatric screening instruments and standardised psychiatric interviews have been translated into the Portuguese spoken in Brazil and validated in the primary care setting in São Paulo (Mari & Williams, 1985; Iacoponi & Mari, 1989).

Only four times have the general medical services in Brazil been screened for the presence of psychiatric disorders. In the first study, Santana (1977), along the same lines as the work of Kessel (1960), reviewed the records of 208 patients who attended a health centre in the city of Salvador. Busnello *et al* (1983) in Porto Alegre, and Mari (1986) in São Paulo, both used the WHO self-reporting questionnaire (SRQ; Harding *et al*, 1980) to screen for psychiatric disorders, although the latter also used the clinical interview schedule (CIS; Goldberg *et al*, 1970). Iacoponi (1990) also employed the SRQ–20 to screen 1502 patients in 38 randomly selected primary care clinics in São Paulo. The prevalence rates for the four studies were 15.0%, 55.4%, 52.3%, and 50.0%, respectively.

It is worth noting that, although most patients consult their doctors with physical symptoms, three of the above rates of prevalence of minor psychiatric morbidity indicated that more than half of the population consulting primary care services in these cities also had a minor psychiatric disorder, whether associated with physical symptoms or not.

In Mari's (1986) report of his survey in three primary care clinics in São Paulo, women in the lowest social class groups were more at risk of having a minor psychiatric problem than the patients in the other groups.

Iacoponi *et al*'s (1989) survey of 'at-risk' drinking in the primary care of São Paulo, reported a low prevalence (5%) of patients who answered affirmatively to more than two items of the CAGE questionnaire for detecting alcoholism. The authors also showed that patients who were young, unemployed and newcomers to this city had a 58% chance of being considered 'at-risk' drinkers.

Psychiatry and primary health care in the city of São Paulo

From the epidemiological estimates described above, it is not possible to determine the proportion of people with psychiatric disorders in the community who are using primary health care services. This is mainly due to the fact that the health services in Brazil do not belong to a unified system. The official primary care network is orientated essentially towards the care of the poorer sections of the population, while the better off can find medical assistance in the INAMPS services or the private sector. The city of São Paulo is used as an illustration of primary health care in Brazil.

Primary health care in São Paulo has shown a slow but continuous development of free medical services since the beginning of the century (Pedroso, 1978; Sposati, 1985), and only in the last two decades has a network of health centres been built to cover most of the urban area (Sauver, 1983).

Several health centres, emergency units and hospitals were constructed in the most deprived and populous areas of the city of São Paulo; their structure followed the model set by the World Health Organization, and financial support was obtained from local and international agencies (including the World Bank). The clear aim was to provide first health contact for the urban poor, since the better-off segments of society were already using medical services from the INAMPS and the private sector.

In the 1950s there were only four health centres in the city of São Paulo, which provided infant and maternal care, together with programmes of immunisation for infectious diseases like poliomyelitis, diphtheria and whooping cough. The figure in 1987 was rather different, and it can be seen that an expansion occurred in two directions: firstly, the number of health centres increased to 320, and, secondly, about 30% of these health centres offered not only infant and maternal care, but also dental care, general medical care to the adult population, specialised care for tuberculosis and leprosy, and even psychiatric care.

Since the beginning of the present decade, one in four health centres (80 out of 320) has included in its team at least one mental health worker – a psychiatrist, a psychologist, or a psychiatric social worker; some health centres have a full mental health team with all these professionals represented (SEADE, 1988). Initially, the role of the mental health team was to give secondary psychiatric care in the primary care premises, i.e. acting almost entirely separated as a team, like the US Community Mental Health Centres. This involved the treatment of major psychiatric problems as well as the follow-up of patients discharged from mental hospitals.

More recently, another role has been suggested by the health authorities, which is the liaison and consultation work with the primary care physicians and other members of the primary care team (Cesarino *et al*, 1985); this is a task that has proved difficult to achieve, basically as a consequence of the mental health workers' lack of experience and training in the liaison role.[1]

---

1. Concerned with this problem, some medical schools in São Paulo have introduced two initiatives: firstly, by extending courses of medical psychology to medical students throughout the six years of medical education, and exposing students to the common psychiatric problems of the general medical practice; secondly, long rotations in psychiatric liaison services and primary care clinics were incorporated to the training schemes of residents in psychiatry.

Level III – Conspicuous psychiatric morbidity

Patients with psychiatric problems who seek consultation in the primary care sector may not have their problems recognised by their doctors. The rate of detection of emotional disorders by primary care doctors is called conspicuous psychiatric morbidity. This issue becomes of special importance when it is known that, in order to properly treat (prescribe psychotropic medication or use supportive techniques of psychotherapy), and refer these patients (to psychiatrists or psychologists), these doctors must first recognise the presence of emotional disorders.

Detection of emotional disorders by primary care doctors in São Paulo

Mari *et al* (1987) were the first to study the rate of detection of emotional disorders by primary care doctors in Brazil. With rates obtained from three doctors, they observed a variation in the detection of emotional disorders that ranged from 10% to 49%; these rates were compared to the scores of the screening questionnaire, and some suggestions were made as to the feasibility and cost-effectiveness of the use of psychiatric screening to help primary care doctors in the detection of emotional disorders in their patients.

In a more recent survey conducted by Iacoponi (1990), 63 randomly selected primary care doctors in the city of São Paulo were asked to assess the presence and intensity of emotional disorders in their patients. The mean rate of detection of emotional disorders was 42.3%, and the variation range was 1–91%. Table 13.3 shows the various measures of detection of emotional disorders obtained for these Brazilian doctors.

TABLE 13.3
Overall view of detection and its various measures, by 63 doctors in São Paulo

Measure	Mean	s.e.	Range
Part A. Minor psychiatric morbidity (SRQ–20)			
SRQ	52.7%	1.7	27% to 80%
Part B. Doctors' Assessments (5-point scale)			
Detection	42.3%	2.7	1% to 91%
Part C. Combination of SRQ–20 and 5-point scale			
Bias	0.83	0.06	0 to 2
Identification index	0.52	0.03	0 to 1
Kappa	0.20	0.02	−0.25 to 0.79
Spearman rho	0.26	0.03	−0.18 to 0.79

The doctors participating in this survey were also asked to respond to various questionnaires which asked about their own characteristics like age, sex, years of medical training, and even personality features and attitudes towards psychiatry and mental health. It was found that the doctors' characteristics that most influenced their detection of emotional disorders were the satisfaction with work in primary care, and whether they also worked in private practice and teaching hospitals. Put another way, those doctors who were unhappy in their jobs, and who also worked in their private practices were least likely to detect emotional disorders.

Level IV – Psychiatric out-patients in Rio de Janeiro: the public and the private

It is estimated that a total of 3.5 million psychiatric consultations were delivered nationwide through the INAMPS in the year of 1986, representing just under 1.5% of the total number of consultations in the same year, all clinics included (DINSAM, 1989). The state of Rio de Janeiro shows a slightly different picture: in 1983 the local INAMPS delivered 861 000 consultations through its psychiatric out-patient clinics, which is equal to almost 3% of the total of 30 million consultations observed in all out-patient clinics in the state (IBGE, 1984).

Whether or not this regional difference is significant is a matter of debate. However, Rio de Janeiro is known as the state with the highest concentration of mental health workers in Brazil: in 1978, half of the 663 psychoanalysts in Brazil were working in Rio de Janeiro; of the 58 277 psychologists currently working in the country, 11 389 (19.5%) were working in this state, which contains about 10% of the country's population.

Psychologists are supposed to provide the bulk of mental health care in this level of services in the community. According to a survey on the characteristics of psychologists (Consello Federal de Psicologia, 1988), those who were working in Rio were mostly female (84%), less than 40 years old (85%), and predominantly engaged in some form of clinical work (64.4%). This clinical work, in the form of psychotherapy, was performed in private offices in 66% of the cases; the orientation of the psychotherapeutic work was overwhelmingly psychoanalytic[2], other orientations like analytic psychology, psychodrama and Rogerian psychology never reaching high proportions. Even more astonishing is the finding that 80% of these psychologists either were currently or had formerly been under a psychotherapeutic treatment themselves.

The sort of care that this professional group can offer and to which section of the population is therefore quite clear: after five years of undergraduate training and then another four to five years spent in expensive postgraduate training in the psychotherapies, they see themselves as liberal professionals, and charge patients according to the need of their expenses and rates of inflation in the country. Needless to say, the great majority of the population is excluded from this sort of sophisticated care.

Psychologists are not alone in this aspiration for private practice. Most members of the medical profession, psychiatrists in particular, follow exactly the same pattern, although there is not as much information concerning this group.

---

2. Including Freudian, Kleinian and, more recently, Lacanian branches of psychoanalysis.

Level V – Psychiatric hospitals

In spite of this general availability of psychiatric out-patient services, it must be emphasised that most of the government attention in the psychiatric sector was still being devoted to hospital care. For instance, in 1981, about 4.5% of the INAMPS' budget was spent on psychiatric services; of this portion, 96% was used to pay for psychiatric hospital services, and only 4% for out-patient clinics (INAMPS, 1983).

After the reforms that led to the creation of the INAMPS, many more psychiatric beds were made available to the population, due to the contribution of the private sector. Following the same pattern as other medical specialties, the INAMPS, instead of creating its own network of hospitals, decided to 'buy' psychiatric beds and services from the private sector.

The characteristics of the psychiatric hospitals in the states of Rio Grande do Sul and São Paulo (and their respective capitals) are shown in Table 13.4. Psychiatric beds in general hospitals are not included in this table, and it is estimated that they account for about 5–10% of the total of beds in both states.

TABLE 13.4
Distribution of psychiatric hospitals in two states in Brazil

| | São Paulo | | Rio Grande do Sul | |
	state	capital	state	capital
No. of hospitals				
public	11	6	2	1
private	105	33	16	6
No. of beds				
public	8100	3904	1765	1611
private	28 347	7607	2049	847
Mean duration of				
hospital admission: days				
public	92	83	131	122
private	80	67	39	41
Percentage occupancy				
public	90	95	90	90
private	91	100	85	94
Beds per 1000 inhabitants	1.2	0.8	0.5	0.9

Of particular interest in this table is the predominance of private beds in both states, and the considerably shorter length of in-patient treatment seen in private hospitals. This is probably due to the 'referral' of chronic (and therefore less profitable) psychiatric patients from the private to the public sector. In one public macrohospital in the state of Rio Grande do Sul, the average length of hospital admission in 1986 was 984 days, much above the rate of 131 days shown in the above table.

This seemingly selective process of public and private hospitals was observed in Salvador; different rates of psychiatric diagnoses were observed in all types of psychiatric hospitals during 1981 (Fig. 13.3) (Almeida-Filho *et al*, 1988).

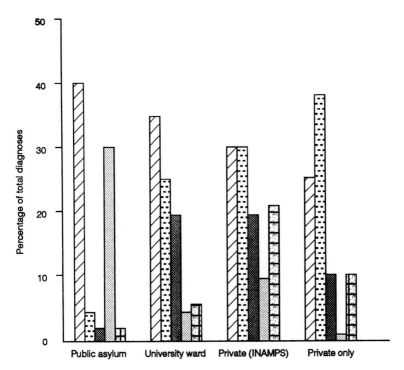

Fig. 13.3. Psychiatric diagnoses (schizophrenia (▨), major depression (▩), neurosis (▨), mental retardation (▨), and alcoholism (▤) in four categories of psychiatric hospitals

The authors that pointed out the fact that psychiatrists in different clinics were possibly not using the same diagnostic criteria, and that this could be partly responsible for the reported variation. However, the number of schizophrenic patients did not seem to vary among the different clinics, whereas the rate of neurosis in exclusively private institutions was ten times higher than that found in public asylums. However, patients with alcohol problems were more often found in private hospitals contracted to the INAMPS than in any other type of institution.

Conclusion

The above description offers some basis for discussion and comparison of the Brazilian case with other parts of the world. At this juncture, some points must be clarified: this report is not intended to be a full and complete picture of Brazil, its health system, and its psychiatric services. In fact, in describing different psychiatric services in a few urban areas, it is far from giving a fair and representative idea of the state of affairs in the whole country. Data concerning the health sector in Brazil, in spite of immense efforts from many people working in this sector, are still scarce, and become even scarcer when one moves away from the relatively wealthy and Western-orientated conurbations.

Finally, psychiatric care in Brazil is very much a reflection of the social conditions around it. The seemingly never-ending divide between affluence and poverty is certainly the most vigorous factor in the shaping of this sector of health care. It also becomes evident that psychiatric services in Brazil, like the rest of the health services, are constantly looking towards the model given by Europe and the United States: medical specialisation, private medicine, a national health service, primary health care, these are all models that come from the more developed group of nations, and are taken as *the* goals to be achieved. In that sense, being a mixture of many different models of the industrial society, Brazilian psychiatric services have very little to offer in terms of fresh and innovative initiatives. On the other hand, it remains to be seen how the psychiatric services of the future will embrace, or perhaps be embraced by, the thus far unofficial system of health care, the only one that is meaningfully available to an unfortunate but still enormous number of Brazilian citizens.

References

ABRANCHES, S. H. (1985). *Os Despossuídos. Crescimento e pobreza no país do milagre*. Rio de Janeiro: Jorge Zahar.

ALMEIDA-FILHO, N., SANTANA, V. S. & MARI, J. J. (1988) *Principios de Epidemiologia para trabajadores de Salud Mental*. Montevideo: PROCSAM.

AMERICAN PSYCHIATRIC ASSOCIATION (1980) *Diagnostic and Statistical Manual of Mental Disorders* (DSM–III) (3rd edn). Washington, DC: APA.

ARGANDOÑA, M. & KIEV, A. (1972) *Mental Health in the Developing World: A Case Study in Latin America*. New York: Free Press.

BANTA, H. D. (1986) Medical technology and developing countries: the case of Brazil. *International Journal of Health Services*, **16**, 363–373.

BASTOS, M. V. (1971) Brazil's multiple social insurance programs and their influence on medical care. *International Journal of Health Services*, **1**, 382–383.

BRANDÃO, M. A. L. (1984) *Médicos e Curandeiros: conflito social e saúde*. São Paulo: DIFEL.

BUSNELLO, E. L., LIMA, B. & BERTOLOTTE, J. M. (1983) Aspectos interculturais de classificação e diagnóstico. *Jornal Brasileiro de Psiquiátria*, **4**, 207–210.

BUSSAB, W. O. (1984) Os médicos de São Paulo: onde estão? *Estudos FUNDAP*, 53–65.

CACEX (CARTERIA DO COMÉRCIO EXTERIOR DO BANCO DO BRASIL) (1988) Estatísticas. *Revista da CACEX*, **23**, 18–26.

CESARINO, A. C., SANTOS, D. N., MACIA, E. V., *et al* (1985) Projeto de ações integradas de saúde mental na zona norte do município de São Paulo. *Revista da Associação Brasileira de Psiquiátria*, **7**, 131–139.

CONSELHO FEDERAL DE PSICOLOGIA (1988) *Quem é o psicólozo Brasileiro?* São Paulo: Edicon.

CORDEIRO, H. (1980) *A Indústria de Saúde no Brasil*. Rio de Janeiro: Graal.

DA CUNHA, E. (1947) *Revolt in the Backlands* (1st edn 1902). London: Victor Gollancz.

DEGLER, C. (1971). *Neither Black nor White*. New York: Macmillan.

DINSAM (DIVISÃO NACIONAL DE SAÚDE MENTAL) (1989) *Prevenção de trantornos mentais, neurológicos e psicossociais*. Unpublished report. Geneva: World Health Assembly.

—— (1987) *Programa Nacional de capacitação da Rede Básica de Saúde para atenção de Saúde Mental.* Brasília: Ministério da Saúde.
DONNANGELO, M. C. F. (1975) *Medicina e Sociedade.* São Paulo: Pioneira.
DURHAN, E. (1978) *A Caminho da Cidade.* São Paulo: Perspectiva.
FRAGA-FILHO, C. & ROSA, A. R. (1980) *Temas de Educação Médica.* Brasília: MEC.
GOLDBERG, D. P., COOPER, B., EASTWOOD, M. R., *et al* (1970) A standardized psychiatric interview for use in community surveys. *British Journal of Preventive and Social Medicine,* **24**, 18–23.
—— & HUXLEY, P. (1980) *Mental Illness in the Community. The Pathway to Psychiatric Care.* London: Tavistock.
HARDING, T. W., deARANGO, M. V., BALTAZAR, J., *et al* (1980) Mental disorders in primary health care: a study of their frequency and diagnosis in four developing countries. *Psychological Medicine,* **10**, 231–241.
HARVEY, R. (1987) *Clumsy Giant. A Survey of Brazil. Economist,* special supplement, 26 April.
IACOPONI, E. (1990) *The Detection of Emotional Disorders by Primary Care Physicians. A Study in São Paulo, Brazil.* PhD thesis, University of London.
—— & MARI, J. J. (1989) Reliability and factor structure of the Portuguese version of the Self-Reporting Questionnaire. *International Journal of Social Psychiatry,* **35**, 213–222.
——, LARANJEIRA, R. R. & JORGE, M. R. (1989) At risk drinking in primary care: report from a survey in São Paulo, Brazil. *British Journal of Addiction,* **84**, 653–658.
IBGE (FUNDAÇÃO INSTITUTO BRASILEIRO DE GEOGRAFIA E ESTATÍSTICA) (1984) *Anuário Estatístico do Brasil, 1984.* Rio de Janeiro: IBGE.
—— (1988) *Pesquisa Nacional por Amostra de Domicílios, 1986.* Rio de Janeiro: IBGE.
INAMPS (INSTITUTO NACIONAL DE ASSISTÊNCIA MÉDICA DA PREVIDÊNCIA SOCIAL) (1983) *Programa de Reorientação da Assistência Psiquiátrica.* Brasília: INAMPS.
IUTAKA, S. (1966) Social status and illness in urban Brazil. In *Behavioral Science and Medical Education in Latin America* (ed. R. F. Badgley), pp. 97–110. Millbank Memorial Fund, USA.
KESSEL, W. I. N. (1960) Psychiatric morbidity in a London general practice. *British Journal of Preventive and Social Medicine,* **14**, 16–22.
LANDMANN, J. (1982) *Evitando a saúde e prevenindo a doença: o sistema de saúde no Brasil.* Rio de Janeiro: Achiamé.
—— (1983) *Medicina não é saúde.* Rio de Janeiro: Nova Fronteira.
LANGENBACH, M. & NEGREIROS, T. C. (1988) A formação complementar: um labirinto profissional. In *Quem é o Psicólogo Brasileiro?* (Conselho Federal de Psicologia), pp. 86–99. São Paulo: EDICON.
LEIGHTON, M. (ed.) (1986) *Brazil.* Amsterdam: Time-Life.
LUZ, M. T. (1978) A saúde e as instituições médicas no Brasil. In *Saúde e Medicina no Brasil* (ed. R. Guimarães), pp. 157–174. Rio de Janeiro: Graal.
—— (1982) *Medicina e Ordem Política Brasileira.* Rio de Janeiro: Graal.
MARI, J. J. (1983) Psychiatric care in Brazil. In *Psychiatry in Developing Countries* (ed. S. Brown), pp. 7–9. London: Gaskell.
—— (1986) Psychiatric morbidity in three primary medical clinics in the city of São Paulo. Issues on the mental health of the urban poor. *Social Psychiatry,* **22**, 129–138.
—— & WILLIAMS, P. (1986) A validity study of a psychiatric screening questionnaire (SRQ-20) in primary care in the city of São Paulo. *British Journal of Psychiatry,* **148**, 23–26.
——, IACOPONI, E., WILLIAMS, P., *et al* (1987) Detection of psychiatric morbidity in the primary medical setting in Brazil. *Revista de Saúde Pública,* **21**, 501–507.
MARTINE, G. (1989) O mito da explosão demográfica. *Ciência Hoje,* **9**, 29–35.
MELLO, C. G. (1977) *Saúde e Assistência Médica no Brasil.* São Paulo: Hucitec.
MONTERO, P. (1985) *Da doença à desordem: a magia na umbanda.* Rio de Janeiro: Graal.
NGOKWEY, N. (1988) Pluralistic etiological systems in their social context: a Brazilian case study. *Social Science and Medicine,* **26**, 793–802.
PEDROSO, O. P. (1978) São Paulo. In *Health Care in Big Cities* (ed. L. H. W. Paine), pp. 194–218. London: Croom Helm.
RESENDE, H. (1987) Política de Saúde Mental no Brasil: uma visão histórica. In *Cidadania e Loucura. Políticas de Saúde Mental no Brasil* (eds N. R. Costa & S. A. Tundis), pp. 16–73. Petrópolis: Vozes.

ROEMER, M. I. (1968) Medical care travel in Latin America. *Medical Care*, 6, 420–423.

—— (1986) The changeability of health care systems – Latin American experience. *Medical Care*, 24, 24–29.

SALLES, P. (1971) *História da Medicina no Brasil*. Belo Horizonte: G. Holman.

SANTANA, V. S. (1977) Trantornos mentais em um centro de saúde de Salvador, Bahia. *Revista Bahiana de Saúde Pública*, 4, 160–167.

—— (1982) *Estudo epidemiológico de doenças mentais em um bairro de Salvador* (Série de Estudos em Saúde no. 3). Salvador: Instituto de Saúde do Estado da Bahia.

—— & ALMEIDA-FILHO, N. (1987) Prevalência de alcoolismo e consumo de álcool em um bairro de Salvador I – variáveis demográficas. *Revista Brasileira de Saúde Mental*, 1, 7–17.

SAUVER, G. A. (1983) O projeto de expansão da rede de serviços básicos de saúde em São Paulo. *Cadernos FUNDAP*, 3, 59–70.

SAYEG, M. A. (1978) A formação do médico generalista e a medicina especializada. *Revista Brasileira de Educação Médica*, suplemento 1, 81–111.

SEADE (FUNDAÇÃO SISTEMA ESTADUAL DE ANÁLISE DE DADOS) (1988) *Anuário Estatístico do Estado de São Paulo 1987*. São Paulo: SEADE.

SEYFERTH, G. (1986) A estratégia do Branqueamento. *Ciência Hoje*, 5, 54–56.

SODRÉ, N. W. (1987) *Brasil: a radiografia de um modelo*. Rio de Janeiro: Bertrand.

SPOSATI, A. O. (1985) *A Secretaria de Higiene e Saúde da Cidade de São Paulo: histórias e memórias*. São Paulo: Departamento de Patrimonio Histórico, série Registros, no. 6.

SSMA/RS (SECRETARIA DE SAÚDE E MEIO AMBIENTE DO ESTADO DO RIO GRANDE DO SUL) (1989) *Informação para o diagnóstico da realidade sanitária em saúde mental para o estado do Rio Grande do Sul*. Porto Alegre: SSMA/RS.

14 Chile: beyond a military interlude – society, health and mental health

RICARDO ARAYA and ROBERTO ARAYA

Chile is located in the south-western part of South America. The country itself looks like a long and narrow corridor with an eastern wall, the Andes mountains, and the Pacific Ocean all along its western side. Chile is a country of every climate and landscape, from a barren northern desert to a southern wasteland of lakes, channels, and glaciers.

Throughout the years, waves of immigrants have come from all over the world to settle in Chile (Europeans, Arabs, Jews, and more recently Asians). The net result is a race as heterogeneous as Chile's geography, with less than 5% of the 13 million population (World Bank, 1989) being native Indians – *araucanos*. Most of the population (82%) lives in or around the three main cities (Santiago, Valparaíso, and Concepción), which receive a constant flow of rural migrants who come to the cities in search of a better life but rarely achieve such a precious dream. Most of these migrants temporarily abandon their families until they secure a place in one of the many shanty towns that form a belt of extreme poverty around the main cities. The recent growth of the agricultural export industry has brought about a new phenomenon. Seasonal workers move to the farms in summer for the fruit harvest and return to work in the cities in winter.

The steady but slow growth (1.7% yearly) of the population has not been matched by increased employment opportunities, particularly in rural areas, although it is improving with the agricultural boom, causing further internal migration (Viel, 1983). The growing elderly population has become a major health challenge; the leading causes of mortality are now 'degenerative' diseases, as in more developed countries with a large proportion of old people (Viel, 1988). The literacy rate is quite high (92%) and it is estimated that 84% of Santiago's population has completed at least eight years of education (Castañeda, 1987).

Chile has traditionally had one of the largest incomes per capita in Latin America. The wealth distribution is not as markedly uneven as in some other less developed countries, a situation which has contributed to the formation of a large and solid middle class. Like many other countries in the region,

Chile has experienced several economic crises since 1970, the latest one in the early 1980s when unemployment reached approximately 30% and a large segment of the population drifted down the social scale. More recently, Chile's economy seems to be recovering, with an annual gross national product (GNP) growth of 4% over the last two years; these official figures have, however, been disputed by the opposition as being artificially inflated for political reasons. Furthermore, there is concern that this economic prosperity has mainly benefited the upper classes. The main criticism of the current economic system is that it lacks social sensitivity and contributes greatly to the gap between the poor and the rich.

Chile was colonised by the Spaniards from 1500 to 1800. The intermingling of Europeans and natives gave rise to a mixed-race society, which achieved independence in 1810 under the leadership of an Irish descendant, Bernardo O'Higgins. Since then, the republic has been ruled for most of its existence by democratically elected governments until 1973, when a military junta deposed the elected president, Salvador Allende. A full analysis of this situation which made Chile famous worldwide is beyond the scope of this paper. It is important, however, to highlight briefly the role played by the Chilean medical profession from before the military coup until the present day.

The medical profession has a long political tradition in Chile, numbering secretaries of state, and members of parliament and senate among its members (Cruz-Coke, 1983, 1988). The ousted president, Salvador Allende, was himself a qualified medical practitioner. The political power and social sensitivity of some medical leaders facilitated the development of a health system of high calibre. In the early 1970s, The Colegio Médico (Chilean Medical Association) supported with general strikes the opposition to Allende's government and postponed a long-awaited rise in consultation fees to contribute to what became known as 'the reconstruction campaign' in 1973–74 immediately after the *coup d'état*. Yet a decade later the financial situation of doctors employed by the state and the overall situation of the nation's health were declared by the Colegio to be catastrophic (Consejo Regional Santiago, 1983). From then onwards the Colegio Médico embarked on a political protest movement which culminated in a leading role in the formation of the "Asamblea de la Civilidad", an opposition organisation representing all sectors of Chilean society, which played a significant role in the return to democracy. The Colegio Médico became an active voice denouncing inequalities in health care, abuses of human rights, and the participation of doctors in the machinery of repression.

Health services

Organisation and financing

Before the arrival of the Spaniards, the Indians had *'hechiceros'* and *'machis'* who looked after the health of their own people. Doctors came with the early colonial expeditions and the very first hospital, 'San Juan de Dios', was founded in 1556 by the conqueror Pedro de Valdivia. But Chilean medicine developed slowly, and it took hundreds of years to equal the advances achieved by Peruvian medicine, which dominated Chilean health services until 1768 (Cruz-Coke, 1988; Medina Cárdenas, 1990). Soon after independence, the nation's health was described as "appalling" by an Irish doctor, G. C. Blest, who had been employed to advise on how to improve Chile's medicine. In 1832, ten years after independence from Spain, the executive committees of the only hospital, the orphans' house, and the elderly hospice, were amalgamated to form La Junta Directiva de los Hospitales y Casa de Expósitos, a centralised committee in charge of all health services (Vio, 1956). The Faculty of Medicine of the University of Chile was opened a few years later (1843) and other hospitals were created throughout the country.

Twentieth century

By the early 20th century, the Chilean state had already assumed some official responsibility for the health of its people. In 1925, social security funds were being used to provide free health services for workers and children, infant milk distribution programmes, disability compensations, and retirement pensions (Romero, 1977; Viel, 1988). The Chilean National Health Service (SNS) was officially founded in 1952 – although already existing under a different name since 1931 – and became the major health organisation in the country, providing over 90% of all hospital beds and employing more than 60 000 workers (Viveros-Long, 1986; Castañeda, 1987). The SNS was supposed to provide preventive care for all citizens, and curative services for working-class and indigent people (65% of population).

A National Medical Service for Employees (SERMENA) was created in 1968 as a government-administered health insurance plan for white-collar workers and their families (20%). Through this programme they could choose their health provider from a list and fees were shared between the government and the user according to a pre-established contract. In addition, the armed forces and the private sector had an estimated coverage of 15% of the population (Viveros-Long, 1986).

This was the situation until the late 1970s. The health care of most of the population was provided by this pluralistic system (see Fig. 14.1), which led however to some organisational inefficiencies and abuses of public facilities by the private sector.

Changes in the last two decades

Following the military coup in 1973, the health system changed substantially. The role of the state in health was redefined in the new constitution of 1980 as having a 'preferential' responsibility to ensure 'free choice' and equal access to a system where all the health care providers would compete to deliver services. Freedom of choice and equality of access became, in theory, the targets of the government but they were never achieved in practice. The poor had little choice but the underfunded state services, while the private sector was mainly accessible to the well off.

In 1979, the SNS was reorganised into 27 semi-autonomous districts with centrally allocated budgets (Scarpaci, 1985). The Ministry of Health was responsible for the drafting of national annual health programmes and policies but its capacity to co-ordinate and ensure the adherence to these programmes was reduced. What was an improvement towards decentralisation became a problem for national planning. Similarly, many rural and peripheral clinics were transferred from SNS management to county or municipal administration, but problems in the way they were financially reimbursed (for their services) and, once again, insufficient mechanisms of control to ensure compliance with central planning, endangered this initiative. Besides, there was no trial period with properly evaluated pilot projects before full implementation took place.

So far, the evidence that the 'municipalisation' programme has changed the efficiency of daily clinic operations is still weak (Scarpaci, 1985; Consejo Regional Santiago, 1987; Jimenez & Gili, 1988). Additionally, some universities and voluntary organisations (for disabled and mentally handicapped children) have retained their government-subsidised services, although on much stricter budgets.

In the 1970s, resources were concentrated mainly in hospital rather than ambulatory care (Jimenez, 1982). The 1980s, however, saw a shift towards increased expenditure on primary care, especially maternal and child programmes, as a reduction in infant and maternal mortality rates became the main health targets (Ministerio de Salud, 1982). The secondary health care level was, as a result, overlooked (Goic & Roessler, 1980; Viveros-Long, 1986). Priority was also given to acute conditions rather than prevention, treatment and rehabilitation of chronic disorders.

All Chilean employees must remit at least 7% of their wages to a government-approved health care system, and Private Health Care Institutions (ISAPRES) (resembling the Health Maintenance Organisations (HMOs) in the United States) were allowed in 1981 to compete for this contribution. Many of these were set up and they fought intensely to attract clients, who also paid monthly fees and, depending on the extent of coverage, a proportion of their curative charges. Their clientele, approximately 1.5 million, is still from higher income groups with low morbidity risk (Castañeda, 1987). Therefore the SNS has not only lost the important 7% contribution of the high-income groups, but it has also become restricted to looking after mainly the high morbidity risk and poorer population (Fig. 14.1) (Viel, 1988; Consejo Regional Santiago, 1989).

In the 1980s, the private sector grew steadily, encouraged by the

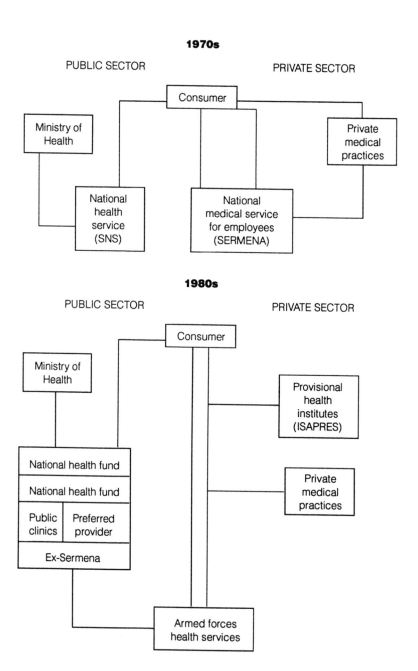

Fig. 14.1. Structure of the Chilean health system in the 1970s and 1980s (modified from Scarpaci, 1985)

government, and funding for health care became more and more the responsibility of individuals. The private sector's (out-of-pocket payments) contribution to the total health expenditure increased considerably as public funding decreased concomitantly (Fig. 14.2) (Razcynski, 1982; Sanchez, 1989).

The Chilean government decreased public health expenditure by reducing capital investments, operational expenditure and medical and administrative personnel (Scarpaci, 1985; Viveros-Long, 1986). The underfunding of the health system has resulted in reduced quantity and poorer quality of services available to the 65–80% of the population who have no access to the private sector.

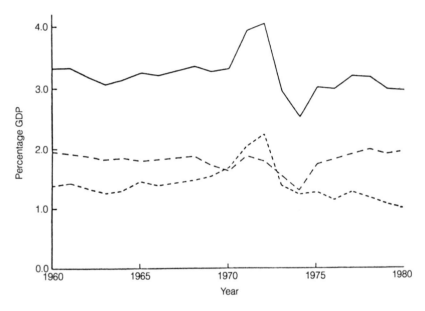

Fig. 14.2. Health care expenditure (total (———), private (– – –) and public (----------)) as percentage of gross domestic product (GDP): 1960–80

The percentage of gross national product (GNP) spent on health is currently between 1.8% and 2.4%, depending on the data used to calculate it (El Mercurio, 1989). The defence budget, on the other hand, has not only grown considerably, but it has also secured by law a high level of allocation for the foreseeable future. Increased budgets do not necessarily bring about equivalent improvements in the health status of a population, but without appropriate funding health priorities cannot be tackled. In spite of all the problems outlined here, the SNS continues to be the main source of health care for most of the population.

Resources

The current structure of the health service is pyramidal within every district. The apex of each regional pyramid is occupied by a large general hospital for the local population within a vaguely defined catchment area. Regional and District Hospitals are still the organisational and administrative backbone of the health service. At a lower level, a network of 'municipalised' primary-care health centres is gradually being developed. The number of primary-care clinics has increased by almost 10 times since 1970 (El Mercurio, 1989).

The number of hospital beds has steadily decreased since 1973. Currently there are 41 833 beds (43 049 according to the government), 3718 private – 54% of which are psychiatric or nursing homes – and 3370 belonging to the armed forces, universities, and other types of hospitals (Jimenez, 1987; El Mercurio, 1989). The average length of stay in public hospitals is two to three times longer than in private hospitals (Jimenez, 1987). Less efficiency, limited resources, and a poorer, iller clientele are possible reasons for these differences.

The number of medical consultations per person per year is approximately 2.4, close to the 3–4 contacts per capita necessary for fulfilment of preventive (and curative) goals in the health sector (Gish, 1990). There is some evidence, however, that certain segments of the population may have more consultations than others, possibly of a trivial nature, hiding the relative lack of attention to other groups in more need (Jimenez, 1987).

There are approximately 13 430 doctors in Chile (Medina & Kaempfer, 1988), with a ratio in the capital of approximately 1 per 800 population compared to 1 per 5000 in other regions. Chile therefore occupies an intermediate position in Latin America in medical manpower (see Table 14.1). However, these data must be looked at with caution. In fact, only 45% of doctors work for the SNS, fewer than 5 per 10 000 people, and the majority are only part-time, spending their remaining time in private work to compensate for their loss of earnings (Ugarte, 1979; Neghme, 1984a; El Mercurio, 1989).

TABLE 14.1
Provision of doctors in some American countries

Country	Year	Population (millions)	Doctors (thousands)	No. of doctors per 10 000 population
Chile	88	13.0	13.4	10.3
Argentina	80	27.9	46.4	16.5
Brazil	80	119.1	101.8	8.5
Colombia	85	28.1	18.2	6.4
Cuba	85	10.0	22.9	22.9
USA	82	236.1	465.0	19.7

(Modified from Passos & Brito, 1986)

Health services personnel, especially medical graduates, have been greatly reduced since 1974 (Medina & Kaempffer, 1982). In 1977, 72% of medical graduates were employed by the government whereas only 13.4% were contracted in 1988 (Consejo Regional Santiago, 1984, 1989). A 20% reduction in the number of students entering medical school has been planned for the next decade (Goic, 1988). This reduction, criticised by some experts, is based on a prediction by a government commission of a 4543 oversupply of physicians by the year 2000 (Comisión de Salud del Consejo Económico y Social, 1987). The unequal geographical distribution and the understaffing of state health services are two major problems in need of solutions.

Private practice has become one of the major sources of employment for newly qualified doctors. However, the supply of doctors for this sector, covering 10–20% of the population, is too large. This has resulted in medical unemployment, low wages, and a justification for reducing the size of the medical force (Acuña, 1984; Neghme, 1984b). All restrictions and regulations for doctors engaging in private practice were abolished in keeping with the free-market spirit. Nowadays, any person holding a recognised medical qualification can work privately in whatever specialty he or she wishes.

It has been estimated that 10% of Chilean doctors currently practise abroad. The temptation to leave is high and some developed countries are short of junior doctors. Unfortunately the training offered in a developed country is often irrelevant and increases the frustration on return. The way forward for developing countries is to establish and strengthen their own local and regional centres (Moodley & Araya, 1990).

The SNS employs approximately 2.5 nurses and 20 auxiliary nurses per 10 000 population. There has been an increase in the number of nursing jobs offered, but it is still far short of matching the yearly output from nursing schools and, more importantly, the needs of the country. Many jobs advertised for auxiliary nurses are vacant because the wages offered are unacceptably low. Average annual salaries for the SNS in 1975 represented 54.4% of their levels in 1970 (Viveros-Long, 1986).

Policies, programmes and indicators

In 1988, the general mortality rate was 6.0 per 1000 population, life expectancy was 71.8 years, maternal mortality rate was 0.41 per 1000 births, the severe malnutrition rate was 0.1%, undernourishment in children below six years of age was 9.1%, and hospital deliveries reached 98.4% (Cruz-Coke, 1988; El Mercurio, 1989). Table 14.2 shows specific causes of mortality.

A large health survey found that one or more forms of chronic disease – hypertension and diabetes being the commonest – affected 10.6% of the population and that 25% of households had a member who had suffered from an acute illness over the previous two weeks (Medina *et al*, 1988). The comparison of this survey with previous ones revealed an increase in the

TABLE 14.2
Main causes of death in Chile (1982)

Causes	Mortality (%)
Cardiovascular	27.6
Malignancies	16.8
Accidents and homicides	12.2
Respiratory	8.5
Perinatal	13.5
Digestive	8.6
Others	12.8

(Source: Ministerio de Salud, 1982)

incidence of chronic conditions in Santiago from 9.8% to 12.9% (Medina *et al*, 1987).

As in many other countries around the world, there are few evaluative data to measure the overall impact of health policies and programmes, and even when data are available, their reliability and interpretation are usually controversial (Etten & Rutten, 1983). For instance, a steady decline in infant mortality since the 1970s, to a rate of 18.9 per 1000 births in 1988, is questionable as an indicator of the effectiveness of recently introduced health policies (Puffer & Serrano, 1973; McKinlay & McKinlay, 1977; De Carvalho & Wood, 1978).

A health index based mainly on mortality rates has been used to reflect the country's health. It shows a steady improvement (the lower the index the better the health) in every region, in spite of wide regional variations,

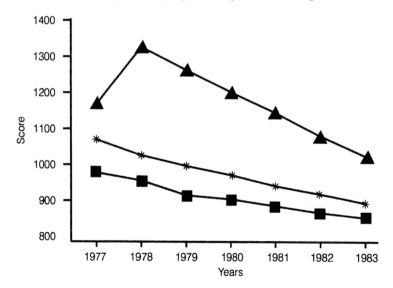

Fig. 14.3. Health index – historical trends for Santiago (—■—), Region XI (—▲—) and Chile (——)
(Source: Tarride et al, 1988)*

since the late 1970s (Fig. 14.3). This approach can be criticised for its excessive reliance on mortality rates. Other important health indicators for a country of intermediate development like Chile such as, for instance, typhoid and hepatitis incidence rates have shown an increase to ''levels unseen for decades'' (Consejo Regional Santiago, 1984).

It should be concluded that the overall status of a given population is multifactorial; many variables are sometimes overlooked, or partial information used and unwarranted conclusions reached (Hakim & Solimano, 1978; Medina & Kaempffer, 1982).

Mental health

Historical developments

The first psychiatric hospital, La Casa de Orates de Nuestra Señora de los Angeles, was opened in 1852 (Roa, 1974). Twenty years later a young psychiatrist, W. T. Benham, was brought from England as the first resident doctor of this institution. He wrote a very critical report and was later dismissed after disagreements with the management board. A decade later he was vindicated by the report of a Ministerial Commission which led to the appointment of P. Montt, later to become President of Chile, as chief administrator (Medina Cardenas, 1990).

Most of the old hospitals were staffed and run by Catholic religious congregations. In 1928, the Open Door hospital, the last of the five Chilean asylums, was created with the aim of rehabilitating chronic psychiatric patients through farming. A hundred years after its opening the Casa de Orates hospital was transformed into the 1200-bed Hospital Psiquiátrico in response to a media campaign denouncing its appalling conditions. Sixteen years later the Sanatorio Putaendo was opened for the transfer of patients from the overcrowded hospitals in the capital, Santiago. Since then a few other small psychiatric hospitals and, more recently, units attached to general hospitals and health centres have been developed.

The many changes, through the years, in what has been considered the best way of providing psychiatric services have resulted in a great heterogeneity in the type of services available throughout the country. In some regions, mental health centres are scattered around; in others, psychiatric services are offered only in units attached to general hospitals, while in other parts of the country, big asylum-like mental hospitals continue to be the only service available (Ministerio de Salud, 1978). Unfortunately, little research has been conducted to compare the efficiency and efficacy of these various systems. A cost–benefit analysis of mental health services and interventions is undoubtedly a complex task. The benefits are not always possible to measure objectively, a problem shared by non-psychiatric services; yet some progress has taken place in other Latin American countries (Climent *et al*, 1978, 1983; Harding *et al*, 1983).

A shift of resources towards the treatment of the acutely ill patients, rehabilitation and discharge of the chronic population, and the development of community care has been slowly taking place. Most of the scarce resources are still being deployed for the care of the old long-stay institutionalised mentally ill. The movement towards a community-orientated psychiatry began many years ago, the main emphasis being laid on prevention, early detection and treatment by general doctors, nurses, and trained community members. Some innovative projects were carried out in the 1960s and 1970s (Horwitz & Naveillán, 1970; Marconi & Muñoz, 1970; Marconi, 1973; Pemjean, 1979). More recently primary mental health care along the lines described by the World Health Organization (1978, 1979, 1981, 1988) has been gaining prominence (Florenzano, 1988).

The provision of mental health services is further strengthened by a few voluntary bodies mainly concerned with mental retardation and alcohol and drug addictions. The relative lack of organisations dealing with mental illness illustrates the prejudice and stigma Chilean society still attaches to it. Intersectoral co-operation has historically been very limited, but prevention campaigns in schools (with no evaluation of their impact or efficacy) are commonplace. The judiciary has resisted a few weak attempts to modify old laws which have, to a degree, increased the stigma of and discrimination towards the mentally ill (Grasset, 1990). There is no mental health act as in the United Kingdom, but patients' rights are supposedly protected by the family and a few unclear paragraphs from the *Reglamento General de Insanos* (1927) (the Chilean mental health act). The prevalence of mental illness in prisons is unknown.

The mental health budget is a reflection of the dismissive approach to mental illness by politicians, other health professionals, and decision makers in general. It represents less than 3% of the total national health budget (Montenegro & Medina, 1977).

Resources

The total number of psychiatric beds, a commonly quoted indicator, was 4500 in 1982. Of these beds, 80% were occupied by chronic patients (50% had been there for 10 years or more) (Medina, 1987). By 1986 there had been a reduction of 800 state beds, mainly chronic but also acute, with the total number left representing less than 0.31 per 1000 population, far below the one per 1000 recommended by the World Health Organization (WHO). The number of private psychiatric beds has, on the other hand, doubled since 1978 (Ministerio de Salud, 1989).

The number of psychiatrists has increased from two per 100 000 to almost four per 100 000 inhabitants in the last decade (Medina Cárdenas, 1983; Medina, 1987; Ministerio de Salud, 1989) – just short of the five per 100 000 recommended by the World Health Organization. However, fewer than one-third of these psychiatrists work for the SNS (Ministerio de Salud, 1978), and of those working for the public sector, almost 80% are in Santiago (Medina Cárdenas, 1983). Most psychiatrists work privately part-time and at least one-third do so full-time. Even if this steady decline in the proportion working for the public sector were reversed there would still be too few to cope with the demand for mental health services (Medina, 1987; Marconi, 1979).

In 1983, there were approximately 45 psychologists, 60 psychiatric nurses, 27 occupational therapists and 501 auxiliary nurses working for the state health services (Ministerio de Salud, 1978). According to the norms laid down in the 1989 National Programme on Mental Health, there should be a multidisciplinary team of a psychiatrist, a psychologist, and a nurse for every 50 000 inhabitants. In other words, the country would need approximately 260 psychiatrists, psychologists, and psychiatric nurses. For chronic patients in rehabilitation, there should be one nurse and two occupational therapists for every 200 patients (Ministerio de Salud, 1989). Since 80% of the 3700 beds are currently being occupied by chronic patients, 15 nurses and 30 occupational therapists are needed to look after the chronic mentally ill population of the whole country.

According to the same programme, psychiatrists should take half an hour to assess new patients, admissions, and emergencies but psychologists could spend four hours for personality assessments. Subacute patients should be reassessed weekly and chronic patients every two months (Ministerio de Salud, 1989).

The problem of understaffing has been partly dealt with by creating stricter filters in the referral process to the specialist. The strategy seems to be helping primary care doctors and nurses to deal with psychosocial problems and reserve the specialist for a few selected cases whose management is difficult. Although the idea is appealing, the implementation of this approach has been patchy. The primary care network is not yet sufficiently developed and health personnel, in general, lack proper training to deal with psychosocial problems, probably as a result of their hospital-orientated education. A recent study found that primary care doctors missed two-thirds of the psychiatric cases detected by short questionnaires. In addition, doctors tended to overprescribe addictive tranquillisers and half of all attenders at a primary care clinic had been on benzodiazepines (Araya *et al*, 1991*b*).

The poor supervision and support offered to primary health care workers does not help to improve their motivation to look after psychiatric cases. Yet some improvement has been achieved: since 1978, short training courses on basic psychiatry have been given to primary care doctors (although, to our knowledge, no proper evaluation has been conducted).

As in most Latin American countries, the active participation of the community is underdeveloped. Community organisations inevitably raise people's political awareness and are a potential political threat to any government. In Chile some community organisations were suppressed and others encouraged, depending on political allegiances.

Extreme poverty may not be the best milieu for any imposed programme of community participation. Campaigns of education which effectively reach the community are still very rare. The balance between active community participation and the state's relinquishing of its social obligations is a difficult one to find but a two-tier health care system in which well-off people consult a doctor while poor people talk to a friend cannot be justified (Ugalde, 1985).

Training and research

There are approximately 300 psychiatric training centres in Latin America (Alarçón, 1986). Chile has nine, five in the capital and four in the provinces (Lenz, 1984). There were approximately 180 trainees receiving training in 1988 (Florenzano, 1988). Most training programmes last three years and follow a comprehensive approach but structure in general is loose and much is left to improvisation.

Instructors are usually part-timers with great devotion to teaching but usually no payment for it. An examination at the end of the training is optional but 20–25% of the trainees sit the exam to improve their credentials (Lenz, 1984). The Chilean Medical Association has created a commission to study the re-introduction of specialty accreditation, which was compulsory before 1973.

Trainees are usually self-supporting financially, and cannot be expected to make a full commitment to the training programme as they need to hold parallel jobs to make their living. Most training used to be sited in psychiatric hospitals, contemporary equivalents of the old asylums but this is gradually changing, and currently trainees are requested to rotate through various posts including: acute and chronic wards, alcohol units, neurology and liaison departments, children's units, and emergency clinics. Some programmes have also included compulsory work with primary care teams in the community.

The teaching of social sciences and psychiatry for medical students is improving but it is still less than desirable in quantity and quality. A recent study showed, however, that the attitude towards psychiatry among Chilean medical students seemed to be slightly better than in a British sample. The worst attitudes were towards psychiatric patients who were seen as too dependent and demanding (Araya *et al*, 1991*a*). This is not to say that medical students are being appropriately trained for their future work as general doctors. On the contrary, too little emphasis is laid on practical psychiatry and it is not surprising that a large number of psychiatric disorders are missed by general practitioners. Nurses' training is even less structured and no formal community psychiatric nursing training is yet available. The use of mental health workers is still in its very early stages.

There are many schools of thought in Chilean psychiatry. The predominant types are the phenomenological and psychodynamic, with the biological school rapidly gaining supporters. The strong psychodynamic presence and, more importantly, the re-emergence of the biological approach, could be explained by the large North American influence exerted upon Chilean training since the 1950s.

The little research available in psychiatry is usually old and hampered by many flaws in method (Salas *et al*, 1980; Medina, 1987; Medina Cárdenas, 1990). Occasionally a study of excellent quality is published, usually in an international journal. There are three psychiatric scientific journals and every so often a paper is published in a local medical journal. Between 1976 and 1980, only 2.9% of the papers published by *Revista Medica de Chile*, the oldest and best-known Chilean medical journal, were on psychiatric topics (Goic *et al*, 1982).

Programmes

Since 1966, the Ministry of Health, through a team led by its adviser, has drawn up national programmes on mental health. An illustration of the isolation in which psychiatry finds itself is the composition of the advisory group which drew up the National Programme of Mental Health in 1989. There were 46 psychiatrists, one public health doctor, one nurse, one social worker, two psychologists, one sociologist, and, a small good sign, 11 general physicians (Ministerio de Salud, 1989).

Recently, some mental health activities have been incorporated within general programmes, e.g. early psychosensorial stimulation for children, and alcohol and drug prevention programmes. Priorities have changed over the years. Alcohol and mental retardation have been consistently regarded as two of the most important areas (Montenegro & Medina, 1977). Epilepsy and psychoses were also included in priorities of the late '60s (Horwitz & Naveillán, 1970). Although nobody would dispute that these are all major problems, it remains open to discussion how best to deal with them, and whether or not other mental disorders and addictions (tobacco and benzodiazepines) should receive more attention.

Where alcohol and tobacco are concerned, the strategies used so far overlook the most effective but politically unpopular measures of increasing the price through heavier taxation and restrictions on their distribution (Royal College of Psychiatrists, 1986; Grant, 1989). The main strategy has nevertheless been concentrated on school educational campaigns whose effectiveness has never been properly established (Horwitz & Naveillán, 1970; Medina Cárdenas, 1983; Medina, 1987; Grant, 1989). Furthermore, anxiety and depression, which constitute by far the most prevalent mental problems in the general population, consume a large amount of health resources (Jenkins, 1985; Croft-Jefferys & Wilkinson, 1989) yet respond to simple forms of treatment delivered by non-medical personnel (Climent *et al*, 1978; Leon, 1984).

The Ministry of Health defined the following priorities for mental health in 1977–8 (Ministerio de Salud, 1978; Montenegro & Medina, 1977):

(a) There should be at least one psychiatric service per region with a multidisciplinary team working in it
(b) Health personnel should be trained to deal with psychosocial problems
(c) The numbers of psychiatrists should be doubled in five years
(d) Alcoholism and mild mental subnormality are priority targets
(e) There should be at least one bed per 1000 population, preferably in psychiatric units in general hospitals
(f) Rehabilitation programmes for chronic patients should be set up
(g) More resources should be made available for repairing psychiatric hospitals.

Ten years later there has been only limited progress towards most of these targets. Most regions have a psychiatric service, but this is usually understaffed and underfunded. The number of psychiatrists has increased, but the employment opportunities for them has decreased. Some rehabilitation programmes with limited resources have been set up but there is little planning on the alternative placement of old or new chronic patients. The training and practical support to primary health care workers has been very limited, and never evaluated properly. The progress on the main targets – alcoholism and mental retardation – is unknown.

There are only 0.3 beds per 1000 inhabitants and most psychiatric hospitals are in a poor condition. Moreover the overall changes in the National Health Service seem to have hampered the delivery of psychiatric care nationwide (Consejo Regional Santiago, 1987). Indeed most of the crude indicators available for mental health show an increase in the prevalence of mental disorders and addictions (Ministerio de Salud, 1989).

Mental health indicators

Given the chronicity of many psychiatric illnesses, discharge rates are comparatively lower than those for other medical disorders. Similarly, because efficacy is measured as cost per case recovered, it too is a misleading indicator in chronic illnesses, although applicable to acute disorders. Ironically, many of the chronic psychiatric patients could live a much more productive and enjoyable life in the community for less than hospital costs if a rehabilitative effort was undertaken and enough support provided (Knapp *et al*, 1990). This would also reduce the length of stay and improve the discharge rates from psychiatric hospitals.

Resources to attempt this strategy are, however, difficult to attract, given the image of psychiatry as a less cost-efficient discipline and therefore a low priority area. Moreover, public health experts have recommended psychiatric hospitals with 1200–1500 beds and general hospital units with 100–200 beds (Medina, 1987). These recommendations should be carefully reviewed before implementation since it is likely that big hospitals engender many undesirable and maladaptive behaviour. Currently, there are only two psychiatric hospitals with 1000 beds or more in Chile (Medina Cárdenas, 1983; Horwitz & Naveillán, 1984).

Even by the misleading figures for psychiatric disorders in Chile, discharges have increased by eight times in 50 years. This rise might suggest a higher prevalence of psychiatric disorders in recent years, or better treatment and outcome with shorter hospital stays for the non-institutionalised population.

The only large general household surveys of psychiatric morbidity carried out in Chile date back to the 1950s and '60s (Horwitz & Muñoz, 1958; Moya *et al*, 1969; Horwitz & Naveillán, 1970; Marconi & Muñoz, 1970), a golden period for mental health research in Chile (see Table 14.3).

TABLE 14.3
Psychiatric morbidity in Chile

Disorders	Prevalence (%)
Psychoses	0.3–1.4
Neuroses	12–20
Alcohol abuse	5–15
Drug dependency	2
Organic brain syndromes	1–2
Dementia	0.7
Mental retardation	1–1.3
Total	22–42.4

(Sources: Horwitz & Munoz, 1958; Moya *et al*, 1969; Horwitz & Naveillán, 1970; Marconi & Munoz, 1970; Ministerio de Salud, 1989)

The prevalence of neuroses, alcoholism, and epilepsy, but not psychoses, was found to be higher in lower social classes. A more recent national morbidity survey, carried out by public health doctors, found a prevalence of only 2.1% for acute nervous system illnesses, but neuroses were the fifth commonest chronic condition (Medina *et al*, 1987, 1988). The low prevalence rate of psychiatric disorders in this study highlights the many problems which need to be addressed to obtain accurate estimates of mental illness in community surveys. Studies of younger subgroups have shown that 15% of primary school students suffer from a psychiatric problem, 10% of adolescents have a drinking problem and 2% a drug problem (Ministerio de Salud, 1989). In a survey of primary school students ($n = 1383$), it was found that one in five were regular daily smokers (Olivari *et al*, 1989). Another survey of high school students revealed that 58% smoked, with 85% of those consuming up to two packets a week (Salas *et al*, 1982).

Psychiatric morbidity in primary care has been estimated at between 15 and 30% (Muñoz *et al*, 1970; Florenzano, 1986, 1987; Medina, 1987);

however, mental disorders constitute only 4–5% of the total number of ambulatory consultations for a given year (Ministerio de Salud, 1989). A recent study of consecutive attenders ($n = 163$) at a primary care clinic in Santiago showed that approximately 50% of this population were psychiatric cases with any of three widely validated case-detection psychiatric instruments, but that general practitioners detected only 34% of them. The main reasons for consultation at psychiatric out-patient clinics were neurosis (40%), personality problems, mental retardation and neuropsychiatric problems (31%), psychosis (23%), and alcoholism (3%) (Ministerio de Salud, 1989).

The mortality due to cirrhosis of the liver in Chile has been found to be twice that in San Francisco and 63 times greater than in Bristol, UK (Puffer *et al*, 1965). More recently it has been estimated that 4–5% of mortality is from hepatic cirrhosis directly connected to alcohol abuse (Lopez, 1985). The mortality from cirrhosis of the liver and suicide combined is 10–20% of that from all causes (Ministerio de Salud, 1989).

Neuropsychiatric problems are said to be the third most frequent cause of invalidity pensions: a total of 398 000 (6.9% of the total) working days were lost for psychiatric reasons in 1985 (Ministerio de Salud, 1989).

Concluding remarks

Mental health has been neglected throughout the history of Chile for many reasons. In addition to those outlined above, others must be noted.

The absence of consensus among mental health professionals about which priorities and needs should be urgently tackled. The various competing psychiatric approaches and the professional and personal interests and rivalries make any agreement fragile. If there is no agreement on priorities, drawing up programmes and policies becomes difficult. There has been some progress, however, in establishing a few flexible nationwide policies and programmes – the need for flexibility must be stressed so that different approaches and interests can be accommodated. This may result in a slower rate of progress but it might be the only way to ensure continuity in the face of political changes.

Stigma and distrust among the public, including the health professions, continue to be a problem which many psychiatrists in Chile fail to acknowledge. The excessive use of jargon and the tendency to give psychiatry a halo of mystery do not create a good public image. Widely used methods of physical restraint, such as 'safe blankets', and the generalised practice of locking hospitals and wards give psychiatry a prison-like status (Horwitz & Naveillán, 1984).

Psychiatrists have had problems influencing decision makers to adopt a wide concept of health. The government needs to be convinced of the importance of mental health and those circumstances, attitudes, and structures necessary for its promotion and maintenance (German, 1987). The relative lack of valid and reliable data to back up arguments for the preferential allocation of resources further aggravates this problem. Nevertheless, there are local and international data which could be used to show the many advances of psychiatry in the last 30 years (Council on Long-Range Planning and Development, 1990).

Some politicians believe psychiatry should be the solution to all the ailments of society. Psychiatrists at times accept this misconception but fail to meet such unrealistic expectations. The belief is then reinforced that mental health is an unproductive area for public investment. Some social problems need to be solved, or mitigated, before health care techniques are useful. As social and political turmoil increases, the number of persons seeking assistance for mental illness will continue to rise.

The 1950s and '60s brought the illusion that mental health issues had become part of the political and public health agenda in Chile but the 1970s and especially the 1980s did not bear this out. It would be unfair to state that no progress whatsoever has taken place, as some improvements – the decentralisation of services, the reform of asylums and primary health care interventions – must be acknowledged. But these limited achievements over the last 20 years must not distract us from assuming responsibility for the task ahead.

'Better mental health for all' needs health personnel, politicians, government, the private sector, and the community as a whole to be active, but many of those who carry the greatest responsibility, such as health personnel, seem to be unaware of this need. Although the WHO produces much sophisticated technical material on mental health, this does not reach many of those who need to be aware of it.

Notwithstanding the need for more cost-effective interventions and more rational use of resources, the government must assume fully its social responsibility by providing enough resources for the improvement of health. The much abused argument that resources are finite, but needs unlimited, must not deter the community from demanding more for health, relative to other areas of state spending. The little international help received is and will always be welcome but we must not wait for it to arrive – there is plenty to be done and to achieve on our own. The time for action is now.

References

ACUÑA, R. (1984) Discurso para el día del médico. *Revista Vida Médica*, **35**, 63.

ALARÇON, R. D. (1986) La salud mental en América Latina, 1970–1985. *Boletin Oficina Sanittaria Panamericana*, **101**, 611–623.

ARAYA, R., JADRESIC, E. & WILKINSON, G. (1991a) Medical students' attitudes to psychiatry in Chile. *Medical Education* (in press).

——, R., WYNN, R., LEONARD, R., *et al* (1991*b*) Psychiatric morbidity, physicians' detection and health service utilization in primary care clinics in Santiago, Chile. (In preparation).

CASTAÑEDA, T. (1987) El sistema de salud chileno: organización, funcionamiento y financiamiento. *Boletin Oficina Sanittaria Panamericana*, **103**, 544–567.

CLIMENT, C., ARANGO, M. V., PLUTCHICK, R., *et al* (1978) Development of an alternative, efficient, low-cost mental health delivery system in Cali, Colombia. Part I: The auxiliary nurse. *Social Psychiatry*, **13**, 29–35.

——, ——, ——, *et al* (1983) Development of an alternative, efficient, low-cost mental health delivery system in Cali, Colombia. Part II: The urban health centre. *Social Psychiatry*, **18**, 95–102.

CONSEJO REGIONAL SANTIAGO (1983) *Algunas consideraciones sobre la salud en Chile*. Santiago, Chile: Colegio Médico.

—— (1984) *Algunas consideraciones sobre la salud en Chile*. Santiago, Chile: Colegio Médico.

—— (1987) *Convención Médica de Santiago*. Santiago, Chile: Colegio Médico.

—— (1989) *Convención Médica de Santiago*. Santiago, Chile: Colegio Médico.

COMISIÓN DE SALUD DEL CONSEJO ECONÓMICO Y SOCIAL (1987) *Requerimientos de Profesionales y Técnicos para el sector*. Santiago, Chile: Consejo Económico y Social

COUNCIL ON LONG-RANGE PLANNING AND DEVELOPMENT (1990) The future of psychiatry. *JAMA*, **264**, 2542–2548.

CROFT-JEFFERYS, C. & WILKINSON, G. (1989) Estimated costs of neurotic disorder in UK general practice 1985. *Psychological Medicine*, **19**, 549–558.

CRUZ-COKE, R. (1983) Los profesores de la Escuela de Medicina y la Historia Política Nacional (1833–1983). *Revista Médica de Chile*, **111**, 380–387.

—— (1988) Political and social history of Chilean medicine: an outline. *Revista Médica de Chile*, **116**, 55–60.

DE CARVALHO, J. A. M. & WOOD, C. H. (1978) Mortality, income distribution, and rural-urban residence in Brazil. *Population Development Review*, **4**, 405–420.

EL MERCURIO (1989) Aumento de gasto en salud pública destacó ministro. Miércoles 13 de Noviembre.

ETTEN, G. & RUTTEN, F. (1983) Health policy and health services research in The Netherlands. *Social Science & Medicine*, **17**, 125.

FLORENZANO, R. (1986) Prevención y tratamiento de los trastornos psiquiátricos y neurológicos. *Boletin Oficina Sanittaria Panamericana*, **101**, 593–607.

—— (1987) La integración de servicios de salud mental en el nivel primario de atención: una experiencia de diez años en el servicio de salud metropolitano Oriente (1977–1986). *Revista de Psiquiatría*, **4**, 191–198.

—— (1988) Formación en psiquiatría y salud mental: avances y problemas. *Revista Chilena de Neuro-Psiquiatría*, **26**, 101–107.

GERMAN, A. (1987) The nature of mental disorder in Africa today: some clinical observations. *British Journal of Psychiatry*, **151**, 440–446.

GISH, O. (1990) Some links between successful implementation of primary health care interventions and the overall utilization of health services. *Social Science & Medicine*, **30**, 401–405.

GOIC, A. (1982) Investigación en ciencias médicas. *Revista Médica de Chile*, **110**, 159–173.

—— (1988) Necesidad de médicos en Chile: una nota de precaución. *Revista Médica de Chile*, **116**, 1077.

—— & ROESSLER, E. (1980) La atención hospitalaria en Chile. In *Desarrollo Social y Salud en Chile* (ed H. Lavados). Santiago, Chile: Corporación de Promoción Universitaria.

GRANT, M. (1989) Controlling alcohol abuse. In *Controlling Legal Addictions* (eds D. Robinson, A. Maynard & R. Chester) London: The Eugenics Society.

GRASSET, E. (1990) Historia de la legislación referente a los enfermos mentales. *Revista de Psiquiatría*, **8**, 411–415.

HAKIM, P. & SOLIMANO, G. (1978) *Development, Reform and Malnutrition in Chile*. Cambridge, MA: MIT Press.

168   *Araya and Araya*

HARDING, T. W., D'ARRIGO BUSNELLO, E., CLIMENT, C. E., *et al* (1983) The WHO Collaborative Study on Strategies for Extending Mental Care, III: Evaluative design and illustrative result. *American Journal of Psychiatry*, **11**, 1481–1485.

HORWITZ, J. & MUÑOZ, L. C. (1958) Investigaciones epidemiológicas acerca de la morbilidad mental en Chile. *Revista Servicio Nacional de Salud*, **3**, 277–309.

—— & NAVEILLÁN, P. (1970) *Primeras experiencias de psiquiatría en la comunidad en Chile. Grupo de trabajo sobre la administración de Servicios Psiquiátricos y de Salud Mental. Publicación Científica No 210.* Washington, DC: Organización Panamericana de Salud.

—— & —— (1984) *Principios básicos de los programas de salud mental y sus proyecciones para Chile.* Universidad de Chile Departamento de Salud Pública y Medicina Social. Chile: Curso de Licenciados en Salud Pública.

JENKINS, R. (1985) Minor psychiatric disorder in unemployed young men and women and its contributions to sickness absence. *British Journal of Industrial Medicine*, **42**, 147–154.

JIMENEZ, J. (1982) Desarrollo y perspectivas del sector privado en salud. In *Desarrollo Social y Salud en Chile* (ed. H. Lavados). Santiago, Chile: Corporación Promoción Universitaria.

—— (1987) Salud Pública 1987: Proyecto Alternativo. *Vida Médica*, **3**, 40–45.

—— & GILI, M. (1988) *Municipalización de la atención primaria en salud.* Santiago, Chile: Corporación de Promoción Universitaria.

KNAPP, M., BEECHAM, J., ANDERSON, J., *et al* (1990) The TAPS project. 3: Predicting the community costs of closing psychiatric hospitals. *British Journal of Psychiatry*, **157**, 661–670.

LENZ, G. (1984) Postgraduate training in psychiatry in developing countries. In *Training and Education in Psychiatry* (eds J. J. Lopez Ibor & G. Lenz). Vienna: Facultas.

LEON, C. A. (1984) Training in mental health for primary health workers. In *Training and Education in Psychiatry* (eds J. J. Lopez Ibor & G. Lenz). Vienna: Facultas.

LOPEZ, A. (1987) Mortalidad por cirrosis hepática, producción y precio del vino en Chile, 1950–1982. *Boletin Oficina Sanittaria Panamericana*, **102**, 346–358.

MARCONI, J. (1973) La revolución cutural chilena en programas de salud mental. *Acta Psiquiátrica y Psicológica de América Latina*, **19**, 17–33.

—— (1979) *La eficiencia del Programa Integral de Salud Mental: Perspectivas asistenciales, docentes y de investigación. Jornados Nacionales sobre Nivel Primario de Atención en Salud Mental.* Santiago, Chile: Ministerio de Salud.

—— & MUÑOZ, L. (1970) Visión general de la investigación epidemiológica en salud mental en Chile. In *Estudios sobre epidemiología psiquiátrica en América Latina* (eds J. Mariategui & G. Adis Castro). Buenos Aires: Acta Fondo para la Salud Mental.

MCKINLAY, J. B. & MCKINLAY, S. M. (1977) The questionable contribution of medical measures to the decline of mortality in the United States in the twentieth century. *Milbank Memorial Fund Quarterly*, **55**, 405–428.

MEDINA CÁRDENAS, E. (1983) Mental health in Chile: current state and perspectives. *Revista Chilena Neuropsiquiatría*, **21**, 77–90.

—— (1990) Panorama institucional de la psiquiatría Chilena. *Revista de Psiquiatría*, **8**, 343–360.

MEDINA, E. (1987) Las instituciones psiquiátricas desde la perspectiva de la salud pública. *Revista de Psiquiatría*, **4**, 129–142.

—— & KAEMPFFER, A. (1982) La salud en Chile durante la década del setenta. *Revista Médica de Chile*, **110**, 1004.

—— & —— (1988) Necesidad de médicos en Chile. *Revista Médica de Chile*, **116**, 389–394.

——, CUMSILLE, F., *et al* (1987) Surveys of morbidity and medical care as a method of analyzing health status. *Boletin Oficina Sanittaria Panamericana*, **102**, 594–605.

——, MARTINEZ, L., *et al* (1988) A population morbidity survey in twelve Chilean cities. *Revista Médica de Chile*, **116**, 476–481.

MINISTERIO DE SALUD (1978) *Políticas de Salud Mental del Ministerio.* Santiago, Chile: Ministerio de Salud.

—— (1982) *Informe del Gobierno de Chile a la XXI Conferencia Sanitaria Panamericana, 1978–1981.* Santiago, Chile: Ministerio de Salud.

—— (1989) *Políticas de Salud Mental del Ministerio.* Santiago, Chile: Ministerio de Salud.

MONTENEGRO, H. & MEDINA, E. (1977) Salud mental en el Servicio Nacional de Salud. Algunos indicadores sobre su situación actual y pautas generales de acción. *Cuadernos Médicos Sociales*, **18**, 5–14.

Chile 169

MOODLEY, P. & ARAYA, R. (1989) Achieving a balance: some unanswered questions. *Psychiatric Bulletin*, **13**, 636–637.
MOYA, L., MARCONI, J. A., HORWITZ, J., *et al* (1969) Estudio de prevalencia de desórdenes mentales en el área norte de Santiago. Comparación de poblaciones de tres niveles socioeconómicos. *Acta Psiquiátrica y Psicológica de América Latina*, **15**, 137–148.
MUÑOZ, L., MARCONI, J. A., HORWITZ, J., *et al* (1970) Prevalencia de enfermedades mentales en el Gran Santiago. In *Estudios sobre Epidemiología Psiquiátrica en América Latina* (eds J. Mariátegui & G. Adis Castro). Buenos Aires: Acta Fondo para la Salud Mental.
NEGHME, A. (1984a) Sobre educación médica y necesidades de médicos. *Revista Médica de Chile*, **112**, 614–624.
—— (1984b) Memoria Anual Academia de Medicina 1982. *Revista Médica de Chile*, **112**, 413–419.
OLIVARI, F., DE LA FUENTE, M. & LOPEZ, I. (1989) Smoking among elementary school children. *Revista Médica de Chile*, **117**, 861–866.
PASSOS, R. & BRITO, P. (1986) Recursos humanos en salud de las Américas. *Educación Médica y Salud*, **20**, 295–320.
PEMJEAN, A. (1979) *El Nivel Primario en Salud Mental, en al Area Sur de Santiago. Jornadas Nacionales sobre Nivel Primario de Atención en Salud Mental*. Santiago, Chile: Ministerio de Salud.
PUFFER, R. (1965) Investigación internacional colaborativa sobre mortalidad. *Boletin Oficina Sanittaria Panamericana*, **55**, 1.
—— & SERRANO, C. V. (1973) *Características de la mortalidad en la niñez*. Scientific Publication No 262. Pan-American Health Organization.
RAZCYNSKI, D. (1982) *Controversias sobre reformas al sector salud: Chile 1973–82*. Washington, DC: Notas técnicas No. 52. Santiago: CIEPLAN.
ROA, A. (1974) *Demonio y Psiquiatría* (ed. Andres Bello). Santiago, Chile.
ROMERO, H. (1977) Hitos fundamentales de la medicina social en Chile. In *Medicina Social en Chile* (ed. J. Jimenez). Santiago, Chile: Aconcagua.
ROYAL COLLEGE OF PSYCHIATRISTS (1986) *Alcohol: Our Favourite Drug*. London: Gaskell, Royal College of Psychiatrists.
SANCHEZ, J. (1989) Radiografia de la Salud. *Cauce*, **215**, 6–11.
SCARPACI, J. L. (1985) Restructuring health care financing in Chile. *Social Science and Medicine*, **21**, 415–431.
SALAS, I., RAMOS, E., PETERS, G., *et al* (1980) Prevalencia del tabaquísmo en alumnos de enseñanza media de las comunas de Providencia y Las Condes. *Revista Médica de Chile*, **108**, 453.
TARRIDE, M., BOSCH, M., MEDINA, E., *et al* (1988) Construcción de un índice de situación de salud: Propuesta metodológica y aplicación. *Boletin Oficina Sanittaria Panamericana*, **104**, 462–469.
UGALDE, A. (1985) Ideological dimensions of community participation in Latin American health programs. *Social Science & Medicine*, **21**, 41–53.
UGARTE, J. M. (1979) Algunas características de la población médica Chilena. *Cuadernos Médicos Sociales*, **18**, 34–39.
VIEL, B. (1983) Población y desarrollo en el contexto latinoamericano. *Revista Médica de Chile*, **111**, 95–103.
—— (1988) Responsibility of the state in health care. *Revista Médica de Chile*, **116**, 61–63.
VIO, F. (1956) *El derecho a la salud en la legislación chilena*. Santiago, Chile: Ed Juridica de Chile.
VIVEROS-LONG, A. M. (1986) Changes in health financing: the Chilean experience. *Social Science & Medicine*, **22**, 379–385.
WORLD BANK (1989) *World Development Report 1989*. New York: Oxford University Press.
WORLD HEALTH ORGANIZATION (1978) *Alma-Ata Declaration. Health for All Series No 1*. Geneva: WHO.
—— (1979) *Formulating Strategies for Health for All by the Year 2000. Health for All Series No 2*. Geneva: WHO.
—— (1981) *Global Strategy for Health for All by the Year 2000. Health for All Series No 3*. Geneva: WHO.
—— (1988) *Eighth General Programme of Work. 1990–1995*. Geneva: WHO.

15 Colombia: beyond the bullets and the drug cartels

FERNAN ORJUELA-MANCERA and
RODRIGO MUNOZ-TAMAYO

Colombia is located in the north-western corner of South America. It is a land of sharp geographical contrasts, extending across 1.13 million km². About half of the country consists of the eastern plains and the Amazonian rain forest. Most of the population live in the mountain and valley areas along the river basins of the Magdalena and the Cauca, and in the low prairies that stretch along the Caribbean coast.

With an estimated population of 30 800 000 (Banco de la Republica, 1989; Proexpo, 1989), Colombia is the third most populous country in South America (*Colombia Today*, 1989). Its population has tripled since 1950. The population growth rate attained a peak of 3.19% per annum between 1951 and 1964. Successful birth control campaigns have decreased its growth to an average of 1.65% per annum between 1973 and 1985 (Corporacion Centro Regional de Poblacion, 1986). Since 1940, the country has experienced a transformation from a predominantly rural society to an urban one; 69% of the population currently live in urban areas. The structure of the population is similar to those of other developing countries, with around 40% of the population under the age of 15.

The ethnic composition of the Colombian population is diverse. Around 48% of the population are *mestizos* (Spanish × Indigenous), 24% are *mulattos* (Spanish × African) or *zambos* (Indigenous × African), 20% are Caucasian, 6% are African and 2% are Indigenous (Ministerio de Salud, 1984).

Despite a central government, there is a high degree of decentralisation, with 15 cities having more than 200 000 inhabitants. Bogotá, the capital, has the largest population (4 200 000 in 1988). Medellín, the second largest city with 2 100 000, is an important industrial and business centre. Cali and Barranquilla also have over 1 000 000 inhabitants (Proexpo, 1989; *Colombia Today*, 1989).

Regional peculiarities and varying degrees of racial and cultural integration have led to four identifiable subcultures. Each of these has its own type of family structure with varying roles for the family members, and different attitudes towards religion, work and money. There are said to be well defined roles for men and women in each subculture (Gutierrez de Pineda, 1958).

Colombia is one of the few Latin American countries which has been a democracy for virtually all of this century. The government is divided into three independent sectors: executive, legislative and judicial. Unfortunately, the presence of the state is still very weak if not absent in many regions throughout the country.

One of the main concerns of successive governments in the last 20 years has been to diversify the economy. The country is the second largest coffee producer in the world and for many years its economy depended on this, but the exploitation of some of its extensive and varied natural resources, as well as the development of a competitive industry provides a firm economic base (*Colombia Today*, 1989). Prudent financial management has allowed the country to resist the temptation to borrow huge amounts of money from the international banks during the 1970s. As a result, Colombia is one of the few countries in the region that is still able to keep up with the payment of its debts. It has had an average rate of growth of 5% per year for the last 20 years and is the only country in the region to have had positive economic growth throughout the 1980s (*Colombia Today*, 1988, 1989; Presidencia de la Republica, 1989). At present, the country exports a wide range of products including oil, coal, coffee, bananas, fruits, flowers; and industrial products such as graphic arts, chemical products, metalworking equipment, and clothing (*Colombia Today*, 1989). As well as diversifying its economy, the country has opened new markets. Most export is to the EEC (35%), USA (28%), Latin American countries (11%), and Japan (6%). There is a special interest in developing trade links with Asiatic and East European countries (Proexpo, 1989).

At the same time, there has been considerable success in reducing the incidence of infant and maternal mortality. In education, primary school enrolment has doubled during the last 30 years and the illiteracy rate of those aged 10 years and over has dropped significantly. The 1981 literacy rate of 78.5% rose to 88% in 1988 (Ministerio de Salud, 1984; *Colombia Today*, 1989).

Despite the economic growth, poverty persists. Wealth distribution remains skewed, with the income of the top 20% being six to seven times that of the bottom 20%. Moreover, impressive improvements in social indicators belie the sharp differences in health and educational status between socioeconomic groups. For example, the birth rate is estimated to be three times higher among the poor, who have shorter birth intervals and higher infant mortality. A high proportion of children from poor communities have no access to any kind of schooling, and the incidence of illiteracy is highest among adults at the lower end of the income stratum (World Bank, 1988).

Available data suggest that approximately 20% of Colombians live below a conservatively defined poverty line. Of particular concern are the prevalence of malnutrition and the high incidence of infant and maternal mortality among these households. Inadequate access to sanitation and safe drinking water perpetuate health problems in poor communities (World Bank, 1988).

As might be expected, the history of dramatic changes in a society with such a skewed distribution of wealth has not allowed peaceful development of the country, which has a long tradition of violence. Through much of the 19th century, the country was torn by civil war between those who favoured a centralised government and those who favoured a federalist one. Virtually every generation of Colombians has lived through a period of conflict.

After 45 years of peace during the first half of this century, civil war erupted again in 1948. The following ten years are known as "La Violencia", a time of relentless bloodshed. This seemed politically inspired by mutual antagonism between the two traditional Colombian parties, Liberal and Conservative. In 1958, a treaty was signed by the two parties, leading to partial peace. After the treaty, conflicts were restricted to certain regions, with the emergence of left-wing guerrillas, 'self-defence' groups, and paramilitary squads of the right wing. During the last eight years the government has attempted several initiatives for peace, offering the guerrillas amnesty if they lay down their arms.

Over the last 15 years, drug trafficking to the USA and Europe has flourished. An enormous and extremely powerful international network has been built under the negligent eye of the authorities in both the exporter and importer countries. The ideological affinities between the drug 'barons' and certain national and international agencies against so-called 'communists', have helped to form an alliance which has received tacit support from some elements of the Colombian society and the US government (Kalmanovitz, 1989; *Sunday Correspondent*, 1989).

The drug network is so powerful that it has become a state within the state, threatening democracy in Colombia (Barco Vargas, 1989; Garcia Marquez, 1990). The drug barons are supported by a national and international network much stronger than the Colombian government, which is too weak to win its declared war on the cartels.

Recently, the government has acknowledged the impossibility of carrying out a development plan without pacifying the country and improving the social conditions of the poor. During the last eight years, the emphasis has been placed on a negotiated peace with the subversive movements, and an improvement in the social standards of the population.

The strategy to fight poverty has three major elements. Firstly, there is the assumption that the country can eradicate poverty only by sustaining a high economic growth and thereby expanding the overall demand for labour. The government hopes to achieve steady gross domestic product (GDP) growth (around 5%) combined with continued prudent internal and external fiscal management. Secondly, the government plans to implement programmes designed to increase productivity and to improve employment opportunities for the poor, through land reform, rural development projects, and education and training. Thirdly, in order to tackle directly the worst aspects of poverty and to achieve a more immediate impact, the government is rapidly introducing some basic-needs programmes, specifically aimed at improving the access of the poor to key social services, e.g. health, education, nutrition, housing and basic utilities (World Bank, 1988). These new policies have resulted in an increase in public expenditure especially in the social sector. For the last five years, health and welfare have taken 25% and education 20% of total public investment. The investment in social programmes attained around US $1000 million in 1989 (Presidencia de la República, 1989).

Despite the efforts of the government, the country may not be able to continue developing at the same rate if the war against guerrillas and drug cartels and the high interest rates on foreign debt go on draining the resources of the country.

Health sector

The health sector of Colombia is subdivided into three subsectors: (a) the official subsector, (b) the social security subsector and (c) the private subsector.

The official subsector

This involves the National Institute of Health, the Institute of Family Welfare, the National Hospital Fund, the National Cancer Institute, and the Department of Health (with 32 Sectional Health Services, 107 Regional Health Units, 497 Local Health Units, 709 Health Centres and 2289 Health

TABLE 15.1
Health provision in Colombia – 1985

Class	Official		Other subsectors		Total	
	No.	Beds	No.	Beds	No.	Beds
Teaching hospitals	11	4817	–		11	4817
Specialised hospitals	44	5213	–		44	5213
Regional hospitals	96	8874	272	14 610	368	23 484
Local hospitals	497	11 586	–		497	11 586
Total	648	30 490	272	14 610	920	45 100
Ambulatory services						
Health centres					709	
Health posts					2289	
Others (mixed)					707	

(Sistema Nacional de Salud, 1989)

Posts). It covers nearly 70% of the population (Ministerio de Salud, 1984). Colombia's Health Institutions, their number of beds, and also the ambulatory health services for the population are shown in Table 15.1.

The social security subsector

This covers the Colombian population working in industries and factories as well as the civil servants of large urban areas (15.8%). This subsector gives health care to the employee, to his wife during pregnancy, and to his children in the first year of life. In some regions of the country, the health care given under this subsector covers the whole family of the affiliate (wife or companion and children under 18, or parents of those single). This subsector also deals with sickness benefits, disability pensions, and life insurance. It is financed by contributions from the employee (33%) and the employer (67%). Between 5% and 7% of the salary of the employees (or as much as 12%, when there is family coverage) goes to financing this health subsector (Ministerio de Salud, 1984).

The private subsector

This not only comprises the private clinics (190), with 8892 beds, but also all the doctors' and dentists' surgeries and the private clinical laboratories. Some pre-paid health care schemes have developed in recent years. It is estimated that between 10% and 15% of the population have access to this kind of health care (Ministerio de Salud, 1984).

Morbidity

As an estimate of general morbidity, a National Health Study with samples of the population from every region in the country showed that over a two-week period, of every 100 persons sampled, 41 felt ill; of these, 24 felt that they needed to be seen by a doctor (11 of whom received sickness benefits) and 0.2 were admitted to a hospital (Pabon, 1980; Ministerio de Salud, 1984).

Important changes have been observed in the trends of morbidity and mortality. There has been a significant decrease in preventable diseases. The general mortality rate has declined rapidly to below 7.5 per 1000, probably as a consequence of the reduced birth rate, the drop in infant mortality, and the increased life expectancy (Ministerio de Salud, 1984). The main causes of mortality are shown in Table 15.2. A number of conclusions can be reached from these findings:

(a) Three of the six leading causes of death during the period 1981–1986 were diseases related to the cardiovascular system.
(b) Enteritis and diarrhoea diminished greatly, coinciding with the

TABLE 15.2
Leading causes of death in Colombia 1981–1986

Causes	1981 Order	1981 %	1984 Order	1984 %	1986 Order	1986 %
Cerebrovascular disease	4	5.7	2	7.8	4	7.1
Ischaemic heart disease	3	5.9	1	8.5	2	8.1
Other cardiovascular diseases	1	7.6	3	7.7	3	7.4
Homicide + accidents	2	6.0	4	6.8	1	9.8
Enteritis + diarrhoea	5	4.6	8	3.0	9	2.5
Neoplasms (cancers)	8	3.2	5	3.8	5	3.8
Other causes	–	67.0	–	62.4	–	61.3

(Ministerio de Salud, 1984; Sistema Nacional de Salud, 1989)

government's efforts on health education, health promotion, and providing communities with drinkable water.

(c) The homicide rate has increased as a consequence of the armed struggle.

(d) Neoplasms are becoming increasingly important as a cause of death.

Health staff

The health sector human resources are summarised in Table 15.3.

By 1982, 80% of health professionals worked in hospitals (Ministerio de Salud, 1984). In the last three years 435 000 health wardens have been trained to work in the community (Presidencia de la República, 1989). Because of an unequal distribution of these professionals throughout the country, some areas have unemployed professionals, while others lack qualified health personnel. The lack of an infrastructure and financial incentives makes it very difficult to get professionals to work in remote places. One way of easing this problem has been the creation of a compulsory social service year for health professionals, which has been operating for the last 40 years.

TABLE 15.3
Human medical resources in Colombia

Human resources	1968	1975	1988
Doctors: total	8650	11 491	23 500
Per 10 000 population	4.3	4.9	8.4
Dentists: total	2740	4123	10 069
Per 10 000 population	1.3	1.8	3.6
Nurses: total	1986	2759	6500
Per 10 000 population	0.64	1.2	2.3
Assistant nurses: total	–	13 539	25 771
Per 10 000 population	–	5.8	9.2
Health promoters: total	–	3293	5310
Per 10 000 population	–	1.4	1.9

(Galan *et al*, 1977; Ministerio de Salud, 1984; Sistema Nacional de Salud, 1989)

Most health personnel come from middle-class families who lack knowledge of the living conditions and social circumstances of the poor.

Budget

The 1981–1982 health budget was US $242.887 million (Ministerio de Salud, 1984), which increased to US $354.996 million for the period 1988–1989 (República de Colombia, 1989). The sources of funds for the health sector come from different areas: national (22.1%), enterprises and affiliates (27.5%), selling services (20%), regional (6.7%), local (1.9%), and other sectors (21.8%) (Ministerio de Salud, 1984). The quality of the services varies considerably from region to region. Generally, teaching hospitals have very high scientific and technological standards, while many health centres lack the minimal equipment to work. The level of integration of the different agencies involved in health care is poor, and there is inefficient use of available resources.

The main health policy during the last few years has been to strengthen primary care. One of the hallmarks of this policy is the active participation of the community in taking decisions and executing programmes. A dilemma health authorities face is how to increase availability of services while at the same time achieving a more efficient use of existing resources.

Mental health services

Mental health services have the same subsectors (official, social security, private) as the general health sector. The official and private subsectors provide 90% of the mental health care in the country (Minsalud, 1986, 1988).

For many years, psychiatry was an isolated discipline practised either in a doctor's office or in huge asylums. Psychiatrists and their patients had no contact with other medical disciplines or society as a whole. Little was done to rehabilitate and reintegrate psychiatric patients into society. There was no national policy regarding mental health except those needed to keep asylum-type hospitals in operation.

In order to improve the situation, and following the recommendations given at The Third Special Meeting of the Health Ministers of South America held in Santiago de Chile (1972), the Department of Health in 1974 created the Division of Mental Health. This body is responsible for planning and executing policies of mental health for the official subsector. From the start, the Division of Mental Health has aimed to gather information to facilitate further planning; extend the coverage of the mental health services in the official subsector, mainly at the primary care level; and develop community approaches aimed at prevention or early detection of mental illness (Minsalud, 1986, 1988). Mental health units, and many

TABLE 15.4
Mental health resources in the Colombian official subsector

	1982	1985	1987
Psychiatric hospitals	13	12	11
Mental health units	15	16	16
Out-patient clinics	27	43	60
Drug dependence units	9	13	85
Farm workshops	1	1	1
Psychiatric beds	3151	2821	2787
Human resources	2200	2587	2605

(Sistema Nacional de Salud, 1989)

out-patient clinics and services for alcohol and drug abuse have been created (see Table 15.4).

The mental health units are located in general hospitals, and their aim is to treat acute cases and return them to the community as soon as possible. In 1986, they represented 12.3% of the psychiatric beds in the country, and the average length of stay was 19 days. Funding for the mental health units is included in the budget of the general hospital to which they are attached.

The out-patient clinics are usually located in general hospitals or health centres. The drug dependence and alcohol units are spread throughout the country – integrated into mental health hospitals or into mental health units of the general hospitals or out-patient clinics. There are plans to create mental health services in areas where at present none exist. For the eastern plains and the Amazonian region, with an extremely low population density (2.3 people per square kilometre), a plan has been developed to cover the population's needs, using the resources of regional health services geographically close to these areas (Minsalud, 1988).

Regarding the traditional mental hospitals, the tendency has been to close some of them and to refurbish and modernise others, e.g. by providing occupational therapy workshops and day-hospitals (Minsalud, 1988). A gradual shift in the ethos of these places towards rehabilitation can be observed. Nowadays, the average stay in these hospitals is 56 days. Unfortunately, the closure of some of these hospitals without the setting up of effective community resources has resulted in many chronic psychiatric patients wandering aimlessly in the streets.

A great effort has been made to provide professionals in the field of mental health with continuous education and training in specific topics such as drug abuse or consequences of natural disasters. International agencies (Panamerican Health Organization/World Health Organization–Convenio Hipolito Unanue) have agreed to supply training and organise research. Several documents, including teaching material, have been published by the Department of Health, and campaigns using the media have tried to raise awareness and disseminate information to the community. Studies in community psychiatry have been carried out in collaboration with several universities;

a Protected Farm Workshop project for the chronic mentally ill and drug- and alcohol-dependent patients is currently under study (Minsalud, 1988).

A considerable effort has been made to improve mental health services in the official subsector, but needs are far from being met. There are huge financial and manpower limitations forcing an emphasis on diagnosis and treatment. Currently, 98% of the mental health budget goes to maintain existing services, leaving only 2% for new developments.

In order to improve the use of resources and decide on priorities, the Department of Health has carried out two detailed studies evaluating mental health resources in each region including public and private institutions (Minsalud, 1986, 1988).

Another agency, also belonging to the official subsector, which is carrying out important work related to mental health is the Family Welfare Institute (ICBF). It was created during the 1960s to protect children and women and to promote their welfare. At the moment it covers 3 250 000 children (around 25% of the population under the age of 15) (Republica de Colombia, 1989). It provides legal and nutritional support, care, and stimulation for poor children. It also gives education to mothers in child care and normal development. Besides the traditional children's homes and nurseries, it has developed, in recent years, day nurseries operated by trained members of the community ('community mothers'), who keep 12–20 children in their homes, allowing the mothers to work. In 1989 there were 46 000 of these nurseries (Presidencia de la República, 1989). This programme has been a model for other developing countries (Republica de Colombia, 1989). Also, the ICBF has special programmes for the mentally retarded or for children with delinquent behaviour. It supports research into the consequences of malnutrition in the development of children and is currently formulating criteria to assess developmental milestones in the cultural context of these children. It sponsors preventive campaigns against drug abuse and keeps a National Centre of Documentation on drug and alcohol abuse. Because of its extensive coverage, the ICBF plays a major role in maintaining and improving mental and physical health in children.

The private subsector comprises 23 institutions located all over the country. They provide an enormous variety of services, which range from asylum-type hospitals to modern short-stay facilities with out-patients and specialised clinics. The private subsector has 2677 beds. Mean in-patient stay is longer (92 days) than in the official subsector. Nothing is known about the number of mental health professionals providing services in private offices (Minsalud, 1988).

Morbidity

A register kept by the Department of Health records details of psychiatric consultation and admission to the official and some of the private psychiatric services (Table 15.5). Interestingly, the number of patients with affective disorders admitted to private institutions is half that of state mental hospitals. One possible explanation for this finding is that the prevalence of affective disorders is higher at the lower end of the social spectrum (Dohrenwend *et al*, 1974; Brown & Harris, 1978; Bebbington, 1985; Der & Bebbington, 1987). But large studies of social psychiatric epidemiology have not been done to test this hypothesis. Another interesting finding is that the prevalence of drug dependence is not as high as might be expected from Colombia's reputation for drug trafficking.

TABLE 15.5

Diagnoses in the official and private subsectors for hospital cases and out-patients in Colombia, 1986

Mental disorders	In-patients		Out-patients	
	Official	Private	Official	Private
Schizophrenic disorders	28.2%	28.3%	18.3%	23.9%
Affective disorders	22.1%	11.1%	9.6%	5.4%
Other non-organic psychoses	7.0%	8.6%	2.6%	–
Neurotic disorders	6.4%	10.0%	17.8%	24.6%
Drug dependence	5.5%	5.5%	2.5%	2.2%
Chronic organic psychoses	4.4%	3.2%	–	1.8%
Paranoid states	3.6%	4.9%	–	2.0%
Epilepsy	3.0%	3.5%	7.4%	7.7%
Drug psychoses	2.7%	3.6%	–	–
Adjustment reaction	–	–	4.0%	4.7%
Personality disorders	–	–	2.4%	5.1%
Mental retardation	2.6%	–	5.0%	3.5%
Other diagnosis	14.5%	17.8%	23.5%	17.3%

(Minsalud, 1988)

Of all the in-patient population, 55.6% of those under the care of the official subsector and 53.5% of those seen by the private subsector are men, a situation very similar to that seen in other parts of the world (Minsalud, 1988). The opposite can be seen at the out-patient clinics and at the private offices of the mental health professionals, where women predominate slightly.

Much attention has been paid to drug abuse, and the results of a screening done in secondary schools in the seven biggest cities of the country between 1974 and 1976 shows the extent of the problem. In spite of abundant drug production, the prevalence of drug problems *per se* is similar to that found in non-producing countries (Minsalud, 1988). However, little attention has been paid to the consequences of the increasing drug trade, such as the increase in the number and the seriousness of the offences committed by adolescents. While, in the past, most adolescents with conduct disorder would be involved only in petty crime, nowadays there are growing numbers of adolescents involved in extremely serious crimes such as armed robbery or murder.

In a country with such a tradition of political violence, the impact of violence on mental health has been denied. There are several theoretical studies that try to explain this process from political, social (Booth, 1974;

Fals-Borda, 1965), and psychological (Leon, 1969) points of view. But there is no systematic research on psychological aspects of violence.

Most of those who attend psychiatric services are in the 15–44 age group (Table 15.6). Mental disorders constitute the fourth most frequent cause of admission to hospital in this age group (Ministerio de Salud, 1984). Usually, general psychiatrists see people of all ages. There are very few specialist facilities for children, adolescents or the elderly (Minsalud, 1986).

TABLE 15.6
Use of mental health services according to age

Age group	Admission	Out-patient
0–4	–	1.4%
5–14	1.0%	12.8%
15–44	80.2%	66.1%
45–59	14.4%	13.8%
60 and over	4.4%	5.9%

(Minsalud, 1988)

Health staff

There are around 1000 psychiatrists in Colombia (3–4 per 100 000 people), which is below the WHO recommendation of five per 100 000. Unfortunately, only 154 (15%) work for the official subsector. Most psychiatrists work in the capital, Bogotá, mainly in private practice. There are few psychiatrists working outside the main cities.

The number of people working in the official subsector has not changed significantly in recent years, largely because of financial constraints. However, the number of services and the population coverage has increased, as shown in Table 15.4, making a much more cost-effective use of the resources. Of the 2605 people that work in the official subsector, 64% are engaged on direct care of patients while the other 36% are administrators. There are 154 psychiatrists (5.9%), 62 psychologists (2.4%), 34 psychiatric registrars (1.3%), 80 medical staff members (3.1%), 13 dentists (0.5%), 16 psychiatric nurses (0.6%), 108 nurses (4.1%), 42 occupational therapists (1.6%), 58 social workers (2.2%), 932 assistant nurses (35.7%), 38 assistant occupational therapists (1.5%) and 39 assistant social workers (1.5%). The number of trained psychiatric and community psychiatric nurses is very low.

Of the 21 medical schools, eight have training programmes in psychiatry. The Psychoanalytic Society and Association have training programmes in psychoanalysis. General training in psychiatry covers a wide range of theoretical and practical approaches, but usually every programme has a field which is emphasised (e.g. community psychiatry, psychotherapies, biological psychiatry (*Revista Colombiana de Psiquiátrica*, 1986)). Training lasts three years, during which the trainees rotate through different services. Most of the teachers have received part of their training abroad (USA, Europe, Argentina and Mexico), allowing the trainee to observe different schools of thought. Most of the training programmes are deficient in child, liaison, and community psychiatry. Some of them are considering extending the training by one year for those wishing to do a subspecialty (social and community psychiatry in Cali or child and adolescent psychiatry and psychogeriatrics in Bogotá and Medellín), but this effort depends on the resources of each university.

Training in psychiatry for undergraduates varies between universities. In general, the focus is on psychiatric in-patients, so that the general practitioner is not trained to detect emotional disorders in his or her surgery. This was shown by Lima *et al* (1989), who found that GPs lacked the skills to detect an emotional disorder in patients who had experienced a severe stress produced by a natural disaster. Other health professionals receive little or no training regarding mental health, and most of their knowledge and skills are acquired in practice when they start their jobs. Several universities have recently started postgraduate training in clinical psychology, neuro-psychology and psychiatric nursing.

One striking feature of mental health care, which also applies to many other countries in Latin America, is the lack of exchange of ideas and cooperation between the different institutions and professionals providing mental health care. There is still a colonial attitude towards new knowledge, as most of the training institutions only look outside the country for updated information. There is a lack of confidence in research carried out locally, with a tendency to be overcritical or dismissive. Some important research has been carried out in Colombia, especially in community psychiatry (Leon, 1976; Climent *et al*, 1980, 1983). Unfortunately, most of this work is better known abroad than in its country of origin. Institutions may have developed original strategies relevant to our own culture, but there is usually a lack of evaluation and dissemination of these important ideas. This failure of diffusion adds to financial limitations and the fact that experience seldom has an impact on mental health policies and makes research very difficult.

Nevertheless, there are clear signs of an improvement in this area. In recent years, increasing numbers of studies have been carried out in the country, covering different aspects of general psychiatry, history of psychiatry and psychoanalysis. Training manuals for health professionals and information for the general public have been published, as well as some textbooks. This constitutes an important step towards the knowledge of cultural particularities that may modify the teaching and practice of psychiatry. Recently, there have been several movements aiming at closer integration with psychiatrists in other Latin American countries which may lead to fruitful exchanges of knowledge and experience, given their cultural similarities and comparable stages of development.

Conclusion

It is difficult to give a global picture of the mental health services in a country with such enormous geographical, economic and cultural differences. We do not know what the psychological sequelae are of the long and continuous turmoil which has changed living conditions so drastically in Colombia.

Although the availability of mental health services has increased significantly in recent years, the country is still far from reaching the needs of the population. It will be a huge task to integrate the available services in the official and private subsectors and to render them more pragmatic and efficient.

Until now, knowledge in mental health has been developed abroad and copied and applied in countries like ours. The need to carry out research of our own and to identify solutions for our own problems should be a priority. Another priority is to learn culturally appropriate ways of dealing with mental disorder.

Acknowledgements

We are deeply grateful to the British Council, who sponsored our scholarships to increase our psychiatric knowledge in the UK, and FOM is most grateful to the Instituto de los Seguros Sociales of Colombia, who also sponsored the time during which this paper was written.

References

BANCO DE LA REPUBLICA (1989) *Colombia. Selected Economic Indicators.* Bogotá: Banco de la Republica.

BARCO VARGAS, V. (1989) Drugs and violence: a threat to democracy. Remarks to the American Society of Newspaper Editors, Washington, DC.

BEBBINGTON, P. E. (1985) Psychosocial etiology of schizophrenia and affective disorders. In *Psychiatry* (ed. R. Michels). Philadelphia: Lippincott.

BOOTH, J. A. (1974) Rural violence in Colombia, 1948–1963. *Western Political Quarterly*, **27**, 4.

BROWN, G. W. & HARRIS, T. (1978) *Social Origins of Depression.* London: Tavistock.

CLIMENT, C. E., DIOP, B. S. M., HARDING, T. W., *et al* (1980) Mental health in primary health care. *WHO Chronicle*, **34**, 231–236.

———, DE ARANGO, M. V. & PLUTCHICK, R. (1983) Development of an alternative, efficient, low-cost mental health delivery system in Cali, Colombia. Part II: The urban health center. *Social Psychiatry*, **18**, 95–102.

COLOMBIA TODAY (1989a) Colombia – basic statistics. *Colombia Today*, **24**, 5.

——— (1989b) Colombia's natural resources. *Colombia Today*, **24**, 4.

——— (1989c) The Colombian economy – 1988. *Colombia Today*, **23**, 10.

——— (1989d) A profile of Colombia's major regions. *Colombia Today*, **24**, 1.

——— (1989e) Colombian foreign trade. *Colombia Today*, **24**, 2.

CORPORACIÓN CENTRO REGIONAL DE POBLACIÓN (1986) *Colombia, Encuesta de Prevalencia, Demografía y Salud*. Bogotá: Corporacion Centro Regional de Población.

DER, G. & BEBBINGTON, P. G. (1987) Depression in inner London: a register study. *Social Psychiatry*, **22**, 73–84.

DOHRENWEND, B. P., *et al* (1974) Social and cultural influences on psychopathology. *Annual Review of Psychology*, **25**, 417–452.

FALS-BORDA, O. (1965) Violence and the breakup of tradition in Colombia. In *Obstacles to Change in Latin America* (ed. C. Veliz). London: Oxford University Press.

GALAN, R., *et al* (1977) *Analisis de Demanda y Oferta Medica y Odontologica para Colombia*. Bogotá: Minsalud.

GARCIA MARQUEZ, G. (1990) The Future of Colombia. *Granta*, **31**, 85–95.

GUTIERREZ DE PINEDA, V. (1958) *La Familia en Colombia*. Bogotá: Universidad Nacional.

KALMANOVITZ, S. (1989) La economia del trafico de cocaina. *Revista Cien Dias*, **6**.

LEON, C. (1969) La violencia in Colombia. *American Journal of Psychiatry*.

—— (1976) Perspectivas de la salud mental comunitaria en Latinoamerica. *Boletin de la Oficina Sanitaria Panamericana*.

LIMA, B. R., *et al* (1989) La detencion de problemas emocionales por el trabajador de atencion primaria en situaciones de desastre: experiencia en Armero, Colombia. *Salud Mental*, **12**.

MINISTERIO DE SALUD (1984) *Colombia, Diagnostico de Salud, Politicas y Estrategias*. Bogotá: Ministerio de Salud.

MINSALUD, DIVISION DE SALUD MENTAL (1986) *Macrodiagnostico de Salud Mental*. Bogotá: Subsector Oficial Directo.

—— (1988) *Macrodiagnostico de Salud Mental*. Bogotá: Subsectores Oficial Directo y Privado.

ORDONEZ PLAJA, A. (1989) Ciencia, tecnologia y salud comunitaria. *Cienc. Tec. Des. Bogota (Colombia)*, **13**, 1–312.

PABON, A. (1980) *Morbilidad General. Estudio Nacional de Salud*. Colombia: Minsalud.

PRESIDENCIA DE LA REPUBLICA (1989) *El Cambio Social: Un compromiso con Colombia. Acciones y Resultados de tres anos de Gobierno*. Bogotá: Presidencia de la Republica.

PROEXPO (1989) *Colombia: A Place for Investment (General Information)* Colombia: Publicar SA.

REVISTA COLOMBIANA DE PSIQUIATRÍA (1986) *Organo Informativo de la Sociedad Colombiana de Psiquiatría*

REPÚBLICA DE COLOMBIA (1989) *Ministerio de Salud. Memorias al Congreso. 1988–1989*. Bogotá: Imprenta Nacional de Salud.

SISTEMA NACIONAL DE SALUD (1985) *Censo 1985 – Avance de Resultados Preliminares (Tercera Edicion)*. Bogotá: Minsalud.

THE SUNDAY CORRESPONDENT (1989) 15 October, p. 12.

WORLD BANK (1988) *Colombia, Social Programmes and Poverty Recuperation: An Assessment of Government Initiatives. Report No. 7271*.

16 Mexico: struggling for a better future

ROWENA RESNIKOFF, SALOMON PUSTILNIK and DAVID RESNIKOFF

Mexico is the only nation of the northern hemisphere where the *"mestizaje"* (mixed race) has assimilated religious and political as well as racial values. Mexicans are guided more by traditions than by principles, more by pragmatism than by ideology. Their preoccupation with the emotional and spiritual aspect of life is evident in their powerful attachment to religion and traditions (Fehrenboch, 1983).

The conquest of Mexico allowed the Spanish to indoctrinate the indigenous people with a sense of inferiority which was then inherited by the *mestizos*, encouraging racism against the pure indigenous people and a special respect for the 'whites'. This phenomenon brought about a sense of self-denigration and insecurity, hidden by a mask of 'machismo' and boastfulness, but behind it there is great warmth and human sensitivity. The extended family is the safest place where emotions can be shown without risk, where unconditional loyalty is taken for granted, and where customs are practised and passed on (Paz, 1968).

The ambivalence Mexico shows towards its native past and its indigenous present is shown by attitudes to the indigenous people who, although they are direct descendants of Mexico's proud history, are today the victims of the worst poverty and discrimination to be found in the country.

There are around 8–10 million indigenous people in Mexico, divided into 56 ethnic and linguistic groups, who speak more than 100 different dialects. Some of them, like the Nahuas, Mayas, Zapotecas and Mixtecas, dominate huge areas of the country. A few of these groups continue to live completely in isolation and have conserved the 'purity' of their religious world, although the majority have incorporated into their lifestyle the characteristics of the *mestizo* world (Paz, 1968).

Since the 16th century, they have suffered slavery, forced conversion to Christianity and devastation of their population by the new diseases brought by the Europeans. Forty-three languages have disappeared since the conquest. After independence, the fortunes of the indigenous people deteriorated, and during the Revolution of 1910 they once again made up the majority of the fighters and the dead. However, their presence in the country today has an influence on the everyday life of Mexican society which is visible not only in the food, the colours, and the language, but also in the traditions, beliefs and behaviour of the Mexican people.

History

Around AD 1300, the Aztecs settled in the centre of Mexico, creating the biggest empire of all pre-Hispanic times. By 1521 the Spanish troops, under the leadership of Hernán Cortés, had destroyed the whole Aztec civilisation. Mexico was renamed "New Spain" and became Spain's richest colony. In a short time the Spanish troops subdued the entire Mexican territory, imposing Christianity and a whole new way of life for the natives. Three hundred years of repression had begun for the indigenous people. The Mexican War of Independence began in 1810. The struggle was led by the *criollos* (offspring of the Spaniards), who were motivated by economic and social forces.

During the rest of the 19th century, internal struggles and foreign wars led to the forced sale of almost half of the Mexican territory to the USA (including California, Arizona, and New Mexico). The 19th century also saw the institution of the Reform Laws which separated the Church from the State, diminishing the economic and political power of the Church. There was also a European-style monarchy for a short period of time, and the longest-lasting dictatorship in Mexican history, the presidency of Porfirio Diaz.

No social, political or economic stability was encountered during those times, and it was not until Mexico's bloodiest civil war – the Mexican Revolution (1910) – that the birth of the present state took place and shaped the Mexican republic of today (Fehrenboch, 1983).

Politics, economics and demography

The Institutional Revolutionary Party (PRI) has been in power without interruption since 1929, giving Mexico the longest period of political stability in Latin America. However, it cannot be said that Mexico has been a 'democracy' in the Western sense of the word, at least until the last decade, during which time there has been an upsurge of political opposition, and corruption at election times has become less obvious.

During the latest presidential election, the PRI was returned with its smallest majority since 1929, and there was much accusation of vote-rigging and election fraud. In 1989 the PRI lost its first state election in its history in Baja California Norte.

Corruption is an inherent factor of Mexican life and the driving force behind the political system in Mexico. Every six years a new president comes to power, and the key figures in the civil service and the bureaucratic system change, breaking potential continuity between governments. Without the security which is offered by a permanent bureaucracy, many of these civil servants feel obliged to make the most of their positions while they can. Corruption is apparent at all levels of the Mexican civil service (Paggett, 1976).

After World War II, the economy, as well as public expenditure, grew very fast. At the same time, the federal bureaucracy expanded dramatically. Currently, the failure of the economic model of the post-war period has driven Mexico into its worst financial crisis since the Revolution of 1910.

Mexico today is actively fighting its current crisis. From a political perspective, this is doubtless an unrivalled opportunity in the history of the republic. As we have seen, the government and party politics that have dominated Mexico in the last years are finally giving way to political pluralism. This signifies progress and a maturing political system, both of which justify a growing optimism about Mexico's future (Riding, 1985).

A national development plan has been created which is the government's response to the increasing need to improve the quality of infrastructure and public services in Mexico.

The geography of Mexico is a great asset, with 1.95 million km^2 of land, abundant natural resources, and both Atlantic and Pacific coastlines. Mexico's road to recovery also benefits from what are known as 'Natural Advantages', which include a domestic supply of crude oil and gas, and low labour costs (CONAPO, 1985). These factors have helped to create an atmosphere of political confidence and social calm which, in turn, has prompted an increased flux of investment capital and substantial industrial growth.

Recent years have shown a dramatic reduction in the rate of inflation. In 1987, inflation was 159%, in 1988 it decreased to 51.7%, and in 1989 it was 19.7%. This is outstanding, especially when compared to other countries suffering from hyperinflation. The most important factor influencing the falling inflation rates, and therefore the stabilisation of the peso (the Mexican currency), is the Stability Pact for Economic Growth (Pacto de Estabilidad para el Crecimiento Económico, or PECE), an anti-inflation programme founded in 1988 and revised by the new government in January 1989. The anti-inflation PECE has been one of the most successful ever. It has been able to avoid many of the pitfalls that have caused other countries' programmes to fail (Financing Enterprises, 1989).

Demographic trends

The population of Mexico is 87.7 million, with roughly 58.9 million people located in urban centres and 28.87 million living in rural areas. Mexico City is the largest city in the world, with a present population of 20.6 million, expected to swell to 24.4 million by the end of the century.

Until 1940, the annual population growth rate was approximately 1% and the total population was about 20 million. By 1970 the growth rate had risen to 3.5%, with a population which had increased by 150% during the same period. During the 1970s a massive scheme was introduced to establish some form of family planning. It reached the upper and middle classes, but in rural areas it was far harder to make any impact. The machismo of the male, in a society which equates masculinity with the number of children a man produces (either within his own marriage or outside it), and religious beliefs were a serious obstacle (SSA, 1989).

This demographic explosion has many implications both for today and for the future. Today, 97% of Mexicans are under the age of 64, and 43% under the age of 14, creating huge demands on housing, education, nutrition, employment and health services. It is estimated that by the year 2000, 62% of Mexicans will be between the ages of 15 and 64, with enormous consequences for employment in a society where 40% of the working population are already 'underemployed' (SSA, 1989).

As we approach the 21st century, Mexico will face a great challenge in the care of the elderly, a challenge which will require many resources not available at present. The birth rate is falling in many areas, due to renewed family planning efforts, but the problems caused by the demographic trends of the past 50 years will continue to have great impact on Mexico well into the next century.

Education

Successive governments have sustained – and financed at extraordinary cost – the principle that education is available to everyone who seeks it (Riding, 1985).

However, the demographic trends already described have put a seemingly insurmountable strain on the resources available and Mexico still has to resolve the quantitative problem of basic education. Total illiteracy is estimated at 15% of the population over the age of 15 and functional illiteracy at 25% of the same population (CONAPO, 1985).

In 1983, over 15 million children (87% of those eligible) were being taught; 47% of these children (75% in rural areas) drop out before completing the obligatory six years of schooling (Riding, 1985).

State education is organised into three levels: primary from age six to 12, which is obligatory for all children; secondary from age 12 to 15; and high school from 15 to 18 years of age. A secondary education is necessary for many jobs in the service sector such as shop assistants and factory work, and is mandatory for most types of technical training. High School education and graduation at age 18 is necessary for entry to university and other professional training schemes.

Many parents make great sacrifices to ensure that their children attend secondary and high school, but socio-economic pressures also work against education. Fifty-one per cent of children enrol in secondary school. School attendance is lowest among Indians, peasants, migrants, and people living in poor neighbourhoods, and there are fewer schools per capita in poorer regions (Riding, 1985).

University education is open to anyone who graduates from high school at age 18. The Autonomous National University in Mexico City (UNAM) is partly financed by the government and is the largest of the state universities. UNAM accommodates some 300 000 undergraduates per year, although the drop-out rate from UNAM and other state-run universities in Mexico City is 69% (CONAPO, 1985).

Because of pressure of demand and oversubscription, many schools and universities have few resources, and maintenance is extremely poor, leading to a substandard environment for learning. Qualified teachers are difficult to find – of UNAM's 26 000 lecturers and professors, one-third have less than two years' experience. They are also extremely badly paid, leading to absenteeism and moonlighting – many teachers have two or even three jobs (Riding, 1985).

In urban centres, and particularly in Mexico City, private education is growing fast. Private schools vary in quality from those which are little better than the government-run establishments to those with facilities and resources on a par with schools in highly developed countries. Many private schools are bilingual, and many are run by religious foundations, chiefly Roman Catholic, although the teaching of religion in schools is constitutionally banned. Today, from medium-level bureaucrats upwards, few people would think of placing their children in a state school (Riding, 1985).

Private universities with facilities far superior to those of the state, and dramatically reduced class sizes, have also begun to flourish in metropolitan areas.

Religion

The majority of Mexicans are Roman Catholic, 93% being baptised into the Catholic Church, and there are strong fanatical tendencies influenced by the colonial past. The separation of the Church and the State was achieved in the middle of the last century and the political power of the Church was broken during the Revolution.

However, the Catholic Church is regarded as a continuous threat to the political bureaucracy, and the government has to move very carefully to control the Church; any strong attack could mean the breakdown of social calm. The Catholic Church is very powerful in its support of the right-wing opposition parties.

Family planning programmes and issues like abortion have been greatly opposed by the Church. However, although abortion is illegal in Mexico, between one and two million abortions are performed each year, and there are about 150 000 deaths annually due to complications and bad practice. Abortion is the fourth most common cause of death in mothers; 60% of beds in gynaecology departments are occupied by women who have undergone abortions. Of these women, 86% are Roman Catholic, 65% are married and 70% already have children (Alba, 1982).

The Church also has its positive side, giving some social stability. The local priests' authority contributes greatly to the unity of the rural communities and poor neighbourhoods (Villegas, 1973).

The Mexican family

The family has survived as a powerful and conservative institution and is very important to political stability. Traditions, and moral and religious values are passed on through the family. The extended family gives a supportive structure to young, old, and orphans. Nevertheless, a number of factors have greatly affected the structure of the Mexican family in recent years. These include:

(a) the demographic explosion
(b) migration to urban areas
(c) illegal migration to the USA
(d) "Westernisation"
(e) diminished religious influence.

With the recent economic crisis and the influence of "Western" values (mostly from increasing contact with the USA), this complicated pattern of family stability is changing. Women struggle for sexual equality and liberation, although this process is slow and so far mainly confined to the middle classes (Riding, 1985).

For the indigenous people and peasants, life has changed little since the formation of the colony. Families are large, and there is no birth control. Children are seen as hands for work. Daughters are expected to work at home and to take care of their younger brothers and sisters (Fehrenboch, 1983).

The Mexican woman is the axis of the family in a society where the phenomenon of illegitimate children, broken homes and absentee fathers is common. Women are expected to act as mothers and housewives, and those who wish to pursue professional careers are subjected to heavy social and family pressures (Paz, 1968).

The problem of abandoned children is very acute in the urban areas. In rural areas an abandoned or orphaned child is usually fostered by a family member, but in the slums or urban areas, an abandoned, neglected, or physically abused child may prefer to have his or her freedom and choose a street life. Many of them gather in gangs living in 'ghettos', and from an early age become addicted to inhalants or alcohol. The government has programmes for such children, but, in reality, few are rehabilitated or offered for adoption to 'normal' families. Most continue to live on the streets of the big cities (Eljure, 1985).

Health services

The health of poor people in Mexico is well below the minimum government standards and more than 30% of the Mexican people are malnourished.

The enormous increase in the population has been caused by a drop in the mortality rate, due to the massive programme of vaccination, and a high birth rate. The government has found it impossible to offer health education and other social services at all.

The unemployment figure is around 13–15%, but 40% more work outside the formal employment sector; for example, washing windscreens at traffic lights, selling chewing gum in the streets, acting as car park attendants, fire-eating, juggling, etc. Eighteen per cent of the population control 55% of the total income. Wealthy people in Mexico have a much better lifestyle than wealthy people in many other countries of the world. On the other hand, the majority of the population live between a state of survival and tremendous poverty.

There is no unemployment benefit, sickness benefit, family allowance, invalidity benefit or old age pension, and the majority of the population do not even earn the minimum salary (approx. £2.50 sterling per day in 1990). Most people are thus unable to feed and house their families adequately, and live in an overcrowded, unsanitary environment which leads to health problems. The extremely poor constitute 11% of the population, 54% live under the minimum level approved by the government, 64% do not receive good medical services, 50% do not eat meat and eggs regularly, and 75% live in homes with no drainage. Up to 75% of adults have not finished their primary education, and there is a chronic lack of housing all over Mexico (SSA, 1988).

The majority of problems related to health in Mexico have their origins in poverty, ignorance, malnutrition, and a deficient health-care infrastructure.

The general socioeconomic registers in Mexico hide the marked differences that exist from one region of the country to another and from one social class to another. Malnutrition is, indirectly, one of the main causes of death and poor health. Two-thirds of the population consumes fewer than 2000 calories a day. The main diet for the Mexican peasant is maize (corn), often made into tortillas, and beans. After the USA, Mexico is the world's largest consumer of Coca-Cola and Pepsi Cola (CONAPO, 1985).

Other health problems have been caused by the contamination and pollution of air, water and land. For example, in Mexico City – one of the world's most polluted cities, the incidence of, and deaths from, chest and intestinal infections is enormous (Soberón, 1988).

The migration from the countryside to urban areas has increased the disintegration of the nuclear family which in turn has stimulated the growth in the incidence of alcoholism – seven million Mexicans are alcoholics. This migration has also increased the number of abandoned children – a large proportion of whom become inhalant addicts (Cornelius, 1975).

Almost half of the population never consult a doctor, even though 30 000 doctors are unemployed. During 1983, 14 000 students graduated from the 52 medical schools throughout the country, but only a quarter of this number were employed in the state health care system (Soberón, 1988).

There is a free market for medicines in Mexico, and it is possible to obtain almost any medication from a chemist without prescription. Most chemists are untrained technicians, but will often give advice on medication for all kinds of ailments. Many Mexicans prefer to take advice of this sort than consult a doctor. Herbal remedies – a custom inherited from the ancient culture – are also very popular.

In rural Mexico, traditional medicine such as witchcraft, shamanism and spiritual healing is still prevalent and provides much of the treatment of the indigenous and peasant population

The leading causes of death in Mexico (in decreasing order of prevalence) are (SSA Statistical Annual, 1989):

(a) Intestinal infections
(b) Pneumonias
(c) Diabetes and its complications
(d) Hepatic problems due to alcoholism
(e) Myocardial infarction
(f) Traffic accidents
(g) Homicides
(h) Neonatal medical problems/Chronic pulmonary diseases
(i) Chronic renal diseases
(j) Pulmonary tuberculosis
(k) Malnutrition.

The health care system

The Mexican health care system is a complicated network of different institutions which offer services in all areas of care. These services are organised into three levels:

(a) Primary care – these services should solve 70–85% of health problems. The main objectives of care at this level are promotion of health, prevention of disease, and detection of initial treatable and chronic conditions. They mainly constitute unsophisticated and low-budget health clinics and consulting rooms, attended by family and general practitioners.

(b) Secondary level – the purpose of the secondary level of care is to solve 10–15% of health demands, those which cannot be solved in the primary care facilities. It is an organised network of hospitals and out-patient clinics with trained doctors in different specialties.

(c) Tertiary level – this level of care consists of highly specialised centres to treat the 3–5% of problems unresolved at the previous levels and to promote scientific investigation, and research and education for high-level specialists.

The health care institutions in Mexico can be divided into three groups depending on the type of population that they serve and the type of financing that supports them (Soberón, 1987).

Firstly, there are institutions rendering services to the general population. There are three major institutions in this group which cover approximately 40% of the population, with government funding in addition to a small fee charged to the patient. Most of the services in this group are provided by the Secretary of Health and Assistance (SSA), but the Institute for the Integral Development of the Family (DIF) offers a wide range of services for mothers and children, including mental health, and the Medical Services of the Department of the Federal District (SMDDF) caters for accident and emergency services.

Secondly, there are institutions providing services to particular groups of workers and their families. The Mexican Institute of Social Security (IMSS) constitutes the most important organisation in this group. Its budget comes mainly from the employers (63%), but employees contribute 20% and government and other sources make up the rest. It provides services at all levels of care for approximately 30% of the population. The Institute of Social Services and Security for Civil Servants (ISSSTE) provides care for most of the civil servants (6% of the population) and it is financed mostly by the government although the patients make a small contribution. There are also other institutions catering for oil workers and the armed forces, who constitute less than 2% of the population (Crúz, 1989; Soberón, 1987).

Finally, the private sector accounts for 20% of the medical facilities in the country and caters for 15–20% of the Mexican population. This sector offers a whole range of services including high-technology medical centres (Crúz, 1989).

Psychiatric services

The mental health of the inhabitants of a country is not distinct from their general health since both depend on the conditions of society, such as economic stability, education, social calm, family integration, employment levels and housing conditions. Severe disruption between man and his physical, socioeconomic, and cultural environment generates tension that is difficult for vulnerable people to tolerate.

Much of the investigative work done in Mexico has been limited to urban areas where the population belongs to one or other of two socioeconomic categories – one which is relatively wealthy and tends to be well established within the cities, and the other which contains the inhabitants of the poor neighbourhoods, who are largely located around the peripheries of the urban areas.

The first group tends to consult health centres with affective disorders, neuroses and psychosomatic problems, whereas the second group contains a higher proportion of people with chronic psychoses, epilepsy, mental retardation and sociopathology (De la Fuente, 1977).

Psychiatric disorders represent a great social and economic loss and hardship for affected people and their families. However, in Mexico these problems have long been disregarded and the insufficient resources available for confronting them have been used for other serious problems such as malnutrition, infectious diseases, the problems associated with the population explosion, and education. While the causes of this lack of regard are understandable, they are not acceptable in a system that proclaims itself the representative of justice and social well-being.

What are the mental health problems in Mexico? It is not easy to talk in quantitative terms, because many figures used are derived from epidemiological studies whose defects cannot be ignored. We are obliged to be cautious, but we can say that, in general, the types of psychiatric disorders that occur in the Mexican population, and the prevalence of those that are most incapacitating, are no different from those of other countries.

A superficial review of the history of care in mental health in Mexico emphasises that, until recent times, public services were limited to providing custody behind the walls of an asylum for severely disturbed people.

Nevertheless, Mexico was ahead of other American countries in considering institutional care for those 'dements' who, badly clothed and malnourished, wandered the streets, or were thrown into prison. The first hospital in America dedicated to the care of these people, the Hospital de San Hipólito, was founded in 1566 in Mexico City by Fray Bernadino Alvarez. Unfortunately the work of this first institution did not substantially influence the general situation. 'Demented' people continued without the help that they needed, kept for the most part in improvised buildings donated by charitable institutions, until the beginning of this century (De la Fuente & Campillo, 1976).

In 1910, an important event occurred. President Diaz inaugurated the building of a new 'general asylum' in the grounds of the Hacienda de la Castañeda in Mexico City. The care given to the inmates of the Castañeda was deficient, but not necessarily worse than in other countries (De la Fuente

& Campillo, 1976). At this time and during the following two decades, some private institutions for the care of the mentally ill came into being and these, along with the Castañeda, contributed to the development of psychiatry as a medical specialty in Mexico.

Between 1960 and 1970, the SSA established a network of 11 hospitals, nine of them outside urban areas, as substitution for the failing general asylum. The nine rural institutions represented a favourable change. Unfortunately, appropriate technical and economic resources were not made available for their maintenance, and over a period of several years of poverty and relative neglect they suffered severe deterioration. The other two hospitals, however, the Fray Bernadino Alvarez and the Juan N. Navarro (dedicated to the care of children and adolescents), have overcome some of these problems and the care of the sick in these institutions has developed to more acceptable levels. Both institutions have played an important role in the teaching of psychiatry (De la Fuente, 1982).

The history of child psychiatry in Mexico goes back to the beginning of the century when a children's ward was built in the general asylum. The first textbooks on child psychiatry were published during the 1940s, and there has been a psychiatric unit in the Children's Hospital since 1947 (Velazco, 1978).

In 1974, a training programme in child psychiatry was developed by the Division of Advanced Studies in the Faculty of Medicine at UNAM. This programme observes the standards established by the Mexican Board of Psychiatry and the World Health Organization for training in Child Psychiatry (López & Katz, 1975).

In 1975, the Mexican Association of Child Psychiatry was founded, and in 1978 the Chapter of Child Psychiatry of the Mexican Psychiatric Association was started. This has resulted in further consolidation of the subspecialty (López, 1985).

Epidemiological aspects

In many countries, psychiatric illness is the principal cause of incapacity in two out of every five 'invalids', and in industrial countries one-third of all hospital beds are filled by psychiatric patients. In advanced countries, as well as in developing countries, close to one-fifth of the total number of people who seek the help of medical services suffer from some form of mental disturbance (WHO, 1978). There is reason to think that the prevalence of psychiatric illness could have increased owing to the increase in life expectancy, the higher probability of survival with mental illness today, and the complexity of daily life and tensions in general.

It is estimated that 1% of the total population of Mexico is affected by a severe disorder and that 10% of people are affected by mental illness at some time in their lives (Organización de Servicios de Salud Mental, 1976). The indices of the prevalence of epilepsy, both 'idiopathic' and 'symptomatic',

TABLE 16.1
Prevalence of psychiatric disorders

Illness	Number affected per 1000 population
Psychosis	10.1–14
Alcoholism	9.1
Mental handicap	12.6
Neurosis	134.0
Epilepsy	3.0

(Source: Cabildo, 1971)

oscillate between 3.0% and 7.3%, higher figures than those given by other countries (Cabildo, 1971).

According to Cravioto (1978), seven of every 100 children in Mexico suffer from severe forms of malnutrition, and one in four has nutritional deficiencies. Although the developmental consequences, both physical and mental, are difficult to quantify, they are undoubtedly severe.

Diverse forms of drug dependency are also difficult to quantify. Nevertheless, marijuana and inhalants are the most frequent forms of abuse, followed by amphetamines and other psychotropic drugs, particularly sedatives and tranquillisers. Consumption of psychedelic drugs, such as LSD and mescaline, is tending to decrease, and cocaine is currently limited to adults of a higher socioeconomic class. Addicts of 'hard' drugs like heroin are found along the northern border with the USA, and one study estimates that there are between 5000 and 8000 heroin addicts in Mexico (Medina-Mora, 1974).

In a study carried out in five cities in the Mexican Republic, of addicts in the age group 18–24 the majority preferred marijuana, and in the age group 14–17 the preference was for inhalants. The ratio of male to female addicts over the age of 14 was 7:1 (Medina-Mora, 1978).

As an estimate of alcoholism, the mortality from hepatic cirrhosis, one of the most frequently used indicators, has not varied in the past five years and is the fourth most common cause of death, with a rate of 20 per 100 000 inhabitants. Between 5.7% and 7% of the population over the age of 14 are alcoholics (SSA, 1989)

The relationship between alcohol abuse and violence, accidents and homicides is very high. According to data from the Department of Biostatistics of the SSA, in 1989, accidents occupied sixth place in the list of general causes of death, with a rate of 39.7 per 100 000 inhabitants. Homicides occupied seventh place, with a rate of 16.5 per 100 000 inhabitants, although in some areas of the country the rate is as high as 84 per 100 000 (SSA, 1989). According to the last formal study, in no less than 50% of cases of violence and in 18% of traffic accidents, alcohol is implicated as the cause (Cabildo, 1972).

The incidence and prevalence of personality disorder and neurosis are difficult to estimate. Another indirect indication of the mental health of a country is the rate of suicide. In Mexico, figures vary between 2.5 and 4.5 per 100 000 inhabitants (De la Fuente, 1982).

It should be noted that data relating to mental health in Mexico are averages – the great socioeconomic and cultural differences among the population are not taken into account. A study by the Institute of Psychiatry, comparing the causes of death of patients at the General Hospital in Mexico City (a public institution) and causes of death of patients in a private institution, concluded that in Mexico it is necessary to distinguish between a "pathology of poverty and a pathology of abundance" (De la Fuente, 1982).

TABLE 16.2
Motives for consultation of psychiatric services and mental health clinics of SSA

Motive	%
Behavioural problems	35
Neurosis	17
Drug dependency	9
Mental handicap	6
No psychiatric problem	6
Alcoholism	4
Psychosis	4
Others	19
Total	100

(Source: Sistema de Información Psiquiátrica. Reporte Interno. CEMESAM, 1979)

The sharp socioeconomic and cultural changes, which result from the migration of families from the countryside to the cities, cause problems in the traditional social support systems, undermine established values, and favour an increase in psychosocial problems, be they alcoholism, drug addiction, or delinquency. Unemployment is one of the determining factors in the violence and delinquency, and conditions of life in the large cities are deleterious to the mental health of the population.

Services and human resources

In 1987, the SSA mental health services comprised 11 hospital units with a total of 4400 beds, and 24 mental health clinics which had recently opened in health centres in Mexico City. Other public or private institutions provided approximately 3300 more beds. Of the total number of beds (around 7700), 57% are in SSA hospitals, 24% are in government hospitals receiving subsidies from SSA, and 19% are in private institutions. Sixty per cent of the psychiatric beds, one for every 5453 inhabitants, are located in Mexico City and the surrounding states, while in the central and southeastern regions the figure is one bed for every 55 315 and 44 115 inhabitants respectively (Pucheu, 1984).

These beds are contained within 18 specialised hospitals throughout the Mexican republic. Two of these hospitals belong to the IMSS organisation and 11 belong to SSA. The remaining five are private institutions. There are also 96 general hospitals which provide minimal psychiatric care, of which five have in-patient facilities for patients with psychiatric problems, and there are 198 clinics and health centres which give psychiatric out-patient consultations (Pucheu, 1984).

It is clear that facilities for the care of psychiatric problems are poorly distributed throughout the republic. It should also be noted that for many years, the conditions that prevailed in psychiatric hospitals did not achieve minimal norms and were in some cases appalling.

However, in 1977, the SSA began a programme to improve care for psychiatric in-patients, and to confront mental health problems in those facilities offering better primary and general hospital health care. In psychiatric hospitals, the programme includes material, technical and administrative help, and the improvement of living conditions for in-patients, including nutrition, clothing, housing, treatment, and rehabilitation. This programme was developed over a period of three years, but was occasionally interrupted due to lack of financial resources.

TABLE 16.3
Distribution of psychiatric beds in the Republic of Mexico

Region	No. of beds	Percentage
Mexico city and surrounds	4787	62
North and central	2390	31
South and southeast	550	7
Total	7736	100

(Source: Pucheu, 1984)

The programme also led to the development of mental health care units in health centres, and the establishment of psychiatric services in general hospitals. Each of these has a team consisting of a psychiatrist, one or more psychologists, one or more psychiatric social workers, and a nurse.

The care of children with psychiatric problems has also been developed in these health centres and children now account for 40% of all consultations. Specific programmes have also been designed for drug addicts, alcoholics and the elderly, and include personnel who are specially trained in these areas.

As in institutions, personnel specialised in the field of mental health – doctors, psychologists, nurses, social workers, and occupational therapists – are scarce and badly distributed, the largest concentration being in urban zones. It is unfortunate that a large proportion of those with training are dedicated to private practice and are reluctant to take up posts in the government-financed hospitals or participate in teaching programmes (De la Fuente, 1976). The World Health Organization recommends a minimum of 5 psychiatrists for every 100 000 inhabitants. Argentina has 4.1 and Costa Rica 3 per 100 000. Mexico has 0.8 psychiatrists per 100 000 inhabitants (Iturbe, 1976).

In 1985, a study was carried out to determine with more accuracy the human resources available in Mexico. The results of this study show a total of 1108 doctors who regularly practise psychiatry in the country. Of these, 905 (82%) are men and 203 (18%) are women; 85 practise child psychiatry, and approximately 170 are psychoanalysts. The rest practise in the field of general psychiatry. Of the total number of psychiatrists, 621 (56%) live in metropolitan areas including Mexico City. The distribution of those psychiatrists who work in a subspecialty is heavily skewed towards Mexico City – 145 psychoanalysts and 73 child and adolescent psychiatrists live in the capital (Fig. 16.1).

Of the 1108 doctors who were practising psychiatry when the study was carried out, 80 (7%) dedicated the whole of their time to working in public institutions, 247 (23%) worked solely in private practice, and 685 (62%) combined both activities. Information was not available on the activities of the remaining 8%. There are 385 psychiatrists who regularly participate in teaching activities. Only just over 10% of all psychiatrists have carried out any documented scientific investigation (De la Fuente, 1988).

With regard to other workers in the mental health field, the deficit is even more acute. Notwithstanding an intensive programme of training that has begun in the past four years, there are only 126 social workers with special training in the field of mental health. The number of nurses is abysmal. In the whole of Mexico there are only 22 nurses with formal training in the management of psychiatric patients. The scarcity of personnel in this area is also reflected in the reduced number of occupational therapists and competent administrators. On the other hand, there are approximately 3000 registered psychologists in the country and thousands more unregistered. Few of these choose to work in the programmes in the government's mental health institutions (De la Fuente, 1982).

What can be done to improve the situation? In the past few years there have been concerted efforts to improve training and co-ordinated activities between SSA, the universities and the Mexican Psychiatric Institute, which have resulted in new courses in which 75 more doctors and 20 more social workers have received specialised training in psychiatry, and 15 psychologists have trained in clinical work.

A new 'paramedical' specialty has evolved recently in Mexico – the mental health rehabilitation technician, whose function is to promote socialisation and therapeutic occupation for the chronically sick in-patient. A total of 76 technicians are trained each year.

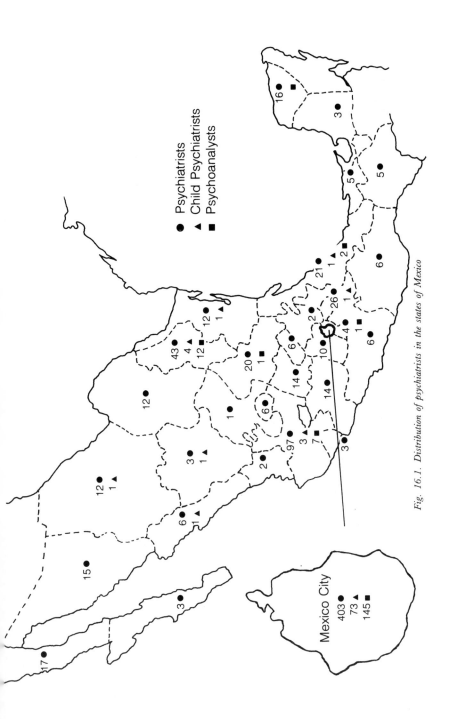

Fig. 16.1. Distribution of psychiatrists in the states of Mexico

Medical education

In 1981, there was a total of 94 321 medical students in 52 medical schools, and approximately 15 000 enter training each year from a total of 35 000 applicants (Soberón, 1987).

In relation to other medical specialties, psychiatry in Mexico has been a late starter both in its human resources and its institutions. Postgraduate training began in 1948 and the psychiatric specialisation course was started in 1950. There are now eight institutions which offer formal courses in psychiatric specialisation, which last for four years, four in Mexico City: UNAM, the Central Military Hospital, the National Institute of Neurology and Neurosurgery, and La Salle University; and four in urban centres in the interior: the University of Guadalajara, the Autonomous University of Guadalajara, the Autonomous University of Nuevo Leon, and the Autonomous University of San Luis Potosi (De la Fuente *et al*, 1988).

The Mexican Council of Psychiatry, the organisation which sets standards for training programmes in psychiatry, holds professional membership examinations, which, although not obligatory for practice in psychiatry, are required for practice in most institutions.

The Mexican Institute of Psychiatry

This is a decentralised public research institution created in 1979 with the following aims: scientific investigation, training of researchers and other health personnel and assessment and monitoring of other official and private institutions in the field of mental health. The Institute has several departments and 294 posts, of which 190 are permanent and 104 honorary. It also has a Clinical Service Study Unit where patients are treated under conditions of controlled observation. The scientific research undertaken by the Institute is classified into three areas: neuroscience, epidemiology and social science, and socio-medical and clinical. During the period 1983–1987, the Institute carried out a total of 187 research projects. These comprised 29% in the Neuroscience Division, 41% in the Social Division, and 30% in the Clinical Division (Soberón & Kumate, 1988).

Conclusions

Mexico is changing rapidly, and new development and stability are being felt throughout its society. Improving the health of the Mexican population is certainly a priority at this time, and efforts are being made in basic areas to fulfil some of the unresolved promises of the past.

Current emphasis is on improving the infrastructure of health care, as well as sanitation, and combating pollution and contamination. In the mental health field, there are active programmes to expand the availability of care to all communities, but much still needs to be done. As the country emerges from a history of deprivation and social conflict, one challenge to Mexico's developing psychiatric services will be to deal with the consequences of this history.

References

ALBA, F. (1982) *The Population of Mexico: Trends, Issues and Policies.* Transaction Press.

CABILDO, H. M. (1971) Panorama epidemiológico de los desórdenes psiquiátricos en la República Mexicana. *Salud Mental,* **13,** 53–63.

—— (1972) Panorama epidemiológico del alcoholismo en México. *Revista de la Facultad de Medicina,* **15.**

CONAPO (1985) *Proyecciones de la población de México y las Entidades Federativas; 1980–2010.* Mexico: Instituto Nacional de Estadistica, Geografia e Información.

CORNELIUS, F. (1975) *Politics and the Migrant Poor in Mexico City.* Stanford, CA: Stanford University Press.

CRAVIOTO, J. (1978) Intersensory development as a function of age stimulation and antecedents of severe malnutrition. *Proceedings of the Nutrition Society,* **22,** 1–24.

CRÚZ, R. C., *et al* (1989) *El impácto de la Crisis Económica de México sobre la Salud y Organización de Servicios de Salud.* CIPS.

DE LA FUENTE, R. (1976) Nuevos enfoques en la enseñanza de la psiquiatría. *Psiquiatría,* **6,** 19–22.

—— (1977) *La Salud Mental en México.* Trabajo Presentado en el Simposio "Los diez grandes temas de la medicina Mexicana", Instituto Syntex. México.

—— (1982) Acerca de la salud mental en México. *Salud Mental,* **5,** 22–31.

—— & CAMPILLO, C. (1976) La Psiquiatría en México: Una Perspectiva Histórica. *Gaceta Médica de México,* **111,** 3.

——, DIAZ MARTINEZ, A., FOUILLOUZ, C., *et al* (1988) La formación de psiquiátras en la República Mexicana. *Salud Mental,* **11,** 3–7.

ELJURE, C. (1985) Algunos aspectos socio-culturales y clínicos en un Hospital Psiquiátrico Infantil. *Salud Mental,* **6,** 3–7.

FEHRENBOCH, T. R. (1983) *Fire and Blood: A History of Mexico.* London: Macmillan.

ITURBE, U. (1976) Los recursos de la salud mental en México al servicio de la comunidad. *Médico Moderno,* **14,** 28–41.

LÓPEZ, M. I. (1981) La formalización del adiestramiento en psiquiatría infantil. *Salud Mental,* **4,** 8–11.

—— (1985) Acerca de la ensañanza de psiquiatría infantil en México. *Salud Mental,* **8,** 17–19.

—— & KATZ, G. (1975) La situación actual de la psiquiatría infantil en México. *Psiquiatría,* **5,** 65–70.

MEDINA-MORA, M. E. (1978) Prevalencia del consumo de drogas en algunas ciudades de la República Mexicana (Encuesta de hogares). *Enseñanza e Investigación en Psicología,* **4,** 111–120.

——, *et al* (1974) *Consumo de fármacos en la población del Distrito Federal.* Reporte Interno, CEMEF.

ORGANIZACIÓN DE SERVICIOS DE SALUD MENTAL EN LOS PAÍSES EN DESARROLLO (1976) *16th Informe del Comité de Expertos de la OMS en Salud Mental. Serie de Informes Técnicos 564.* Geneva.

PAGGETT, V. (1976) *The Mexican Political System.* Houghton Mifflin.

PAZ, O. (1968) *El Laberinto de la Soledad.* Mexico Fondo de Cultura Económica.

PUCHEU, C. (1984) Panorama actual de la psiquiatría y la salud mental en México. *Salud Mental,* **7.**

RIDING, A. (1985) *Vecinos Distantes* (Ed. Joaquín M. Ortiz). México: Distant Neighbors Vintage Books.

Soberón, G. (1985) *Hacia un Sistema Nacional de Salud y Seguridad Social.* México: UNAM.
—— (1987) El cambio estructural en salud''. *Salud Pública de México,* **29**.
—— & Kumate, J. (1988) *La Salud en México. Testimonios 1988 I.-IV.* Mexico: Fondo de Cultura Económica.
SSA (1988) *Encuesta Nacional de Salud.* México: Secretaria Salubridad Asistencia.
—— (1989) *Anuario Estadístico, 1989.* Mexico: Subsecretaria de Planeación y Dirección General de Estadística.
Velasco, A. (1978) *La Historia de la Psiquiatría Infantil en México. Primer Congreso de Psiquiatría Infantil, Guadalajara, 1976.* Mexico: Monografías de la AMPI.
Villegas, C. (1973) *Historia Moderna de México.* El Colegio de México.
WHO (1978) *Medium-Term Mental Health Programme 1975-1982. Interim Report.* Geneva: WHO.
—— (1986) *Basic Data, Mexico.* Geneva: WHO.

VI. International lessons

17 International lessons: an overview

RICARDO ARAYA and LOUIS APPLEBY

What makes "Health for all by the year 2000" an ingenious ideal is also what makes it an easy slogan. It is unimpeachable as an expression of intent, and so can act as a camouflage for inactivity. The countries represented in the preceding chapters are supporters of "Health For All" and many are making important progress towards that goal. But the obstructions that stand in the way are as varied as the routes to bringing it about.

Health is the end product of a complex equation, incorporating economics, politics, religion, tradition, ethnicity, and geography, all interacting and competing. In Korea, for instance, ancient traditions and cultural ties has maintained the stigma attached to mental illness, so diminishing the impact of a well-off health care system. In Colombia, where to mention culture includes going for your gun, the politics of drug trading has helped make homicide a major cause of death, and violence a major challenge to medicine.

Resources – in themselves neither the problem nor the solution

Throughout this book there are examples of how the health of nations around the world is moulded by this complexity of factors, although the mixture is different in each case. You should no more expect the health of two countries to be the same as expect to deal the same hand from two shuffled packs of cards. Yet there are cross-cultural similarities, based on the universal nature of the principles of health care themselves, which do not change from Mali to Manhattan. Population needs are identified, services designed, and resources, both financial and human, deployed. It is this similarity that makes comparisons worthwhile. Such comparisons point to a striking common thread: the inadequacy of resources, particularly money, to match the perceived health need. The most prominent common theme of transcultural psychiatry appears to be the scarcity of resources.

But there is much more to lack of resources than simple scarcity. The shortage is more pronounced in the less-developed world as it struggles to break away from the vicious circle of poverty and ill-health. Poverty makes people sick and increases health need; in doing so it widens the gap between need and supply. Proportionate inequalities seem to be wider when overall resources are limited.

In many developing countries, these few resources are concentrated in urban settings. The rapidly growing cities of, for example, Mexico, grow faster still because of their advantages in jobs and services, with the result that the urban–rural divide, a health care phenomenon as much as a sociological one, becomes more entrenched. This may be particularly true of Brazil and India, where territorial size makes service delivery to remote or rural areas more problematic, and, by thus contributing to regional inequalities, encourages further migration.

But even relatively wealthy countries, such as Korea and Saudi Arabia, have neither achieved equivalent riches in health service development, nor designed services free of inequality. In European countries also, regional variations in wealth, and therefore health and health care, present comparable regional disparities. Italy provides the most striking example, the relative failure of some regions to achieve the targets of the psychiatric reform movement being due, some argue, to an absence of cash for community-based facilities rather than to flaws in the underlying political philosophy.

So the insufficiency of resources is itself only part of the story; as important is its interaction with the inequality it first helps to create. The result of that interaction is a centralised health care system and the success of the Alma-Ata Declaration will depend on how far decentralisation goes.

Centralisation applies to manpower as much as money, both in developed and developing countries, although the people shortage is more acute in the developing world because of the overall scarcity of skill. The size of the problem may not be noticeable when only the ratio of professionals to population is examined, but it becomes more obvious when the number of professionals employed by the state health system – which is responsible in most parts of the world for the treatment of most of the population – is studied. In spite of manpower shortages, there is unemployment among doctors in many countries, notably Mexico and Spain. Elsewhere a large proportion work privately in cities. Even where there is a satisfactory doctor:population ratio, as in Libya, the number of doctors entering psychiatry may be disproportionately low.

Doctors, however, are only one kind of skilled person. The training of village health workers to deliver basic services, including psychiatry, seems to be spreading. It is especially advanced in Thailand and India, and forms the base of a pyramidal referral system in Zimbabwe. Chile and Brazil, on the other hand, have found political barriers can block the devolution of care towards the community.

The additional financial challenge of defining priorities is influenced by many considerations, including epidemiological information, public pressure, popular beliefs, and, most of all, urgent needs. For psychiatry, particularly in the developing world, there is a disturbing question about priorities: how can mental health compete with malnutrition or maternal mortality? But it may be misguided to attempt an answer and better to address a different question: how can mental health *avoid* competing with such pressing problems? Or, put another way, how can psychiatry prove it has a place in an integrated system of health care? Malnutrition can cause organic psychiatric disorders; maternal death and morbidity have important psychosocial causes and sequelae; mental health is not a separate subject. One area where mental and physical health currently mix is the emerging catastrophe of AIDS and HIV infection, which poses its greatest threat in African countries such as Zimbabwe that can least afford a new epidemic.

In some places, the priorities are not what would be guessed from the popular image. In Saudi Arabia, a religious ban on alcohol does not mean alcohol-related disorders do not occur. In Colombia it might have been predicted that drug addiction would be widespread, but it does not seem to be a target for immediate intervention.

Politics and conflict

The social turmoil caused by internal and external wars slows down progress towards health for all at a time when health care may be at its most valuable. Spain, Chile, Brazil and Somalia have endured military dictatorships which have deliberately impeded community participation in health as in other aspects of life, viewing it as potentially subversive.

Spain has now rebounded from political oppression and its throwing off of the fascist system of centralised power, one which crushed regional autonomy, has had its parallel in medical care. Now, in health as in government, devolution is the order of the day.

Somalia's recent experience of a brutal civil war has led thousands of civilians to flee to Ethiopia and the UK. Refugees and other migrants, now a common feature of politics, are a group with a unique experience and particular needs. Many arrive at their destination having been tortured and after losing families and possessions. The mental health impact of what they endure has become a vital subject for study – it may be lessened or made worse by the response of the host society, which may choose to offer a culture-sensitive service or to marginalise its refugees as a racial minority in living conditions which add to their misery. There is a poignant aside in the account of Somalis who settle in the UK: never having faced racism, the refugees find it inexplicable.

For the Palestinians, occupation and ghetto life have proved medically harmful. Health care has suffered, family ties have been strained, and mental health has deteriorated. But it appears that the Intifada has reversed the social disintegration and its psychiatric consequences, as Émile Durkheim would have expected.

Even in the absence of conflict, politics can directly affect the practice of psychiatry as well as mental illness. When, for example, the leftist parties in Italy promoted the radical psychiatric reform, it was as part of a wider political movement. Through skilful lobbying, psychiatry was transformed, but the result was disastrous – lack of funds was part of the problem, overconcern with the theory of institutions was another, and failure to take account of patients' needs was a third. The result was the rejection of the mentally ill.

In the UK, political ideology appears set to transform the NHS almost as radically and the same failings are there – poor resources, overconcern with the theory of the market, and failure to take account of patients' needs. Can an increase in stigma be far behind?

Stigma

The second common transcultural theme, after lack of resources, is stigma. It has affected the treatment of individuals in countries as far apart as Zimbabwe and Korea, compounded the policy failure of Italy and contributed to the low priority for resources in almost every part of the world. It is a facet of human behaviour as fundamental and universal as mental illness itself and infects patients and their carers alike. It is not simply a product of ignorance, but also of superstition, fear and helplessness. If there were no other reason for the integration of mental health with the rest of health, for the training of primary care personnel, whether general practitioners or village workers, to manage mental illness, and for the inclusion of health education in the list of primary care priorities, stigma alone would be sufficient. A decentralising policy, if backed up by a devolved system of care, is an attack on stigma, just as Italian deinstitutionalisation inadvertently enhanced it.

Tradition and religion

The influence of religion on health is most clearly seen where religion is strongest within the national culture. One illustration is the case of Mexico where high maternal mortality and abortion exist beside tight restrictions on contraception, imposed by the Roman Catholic Church. In Saudi Arabia, the Islamic suppression of alcohol use has permitted the suppression of awareness of its abuse, although this may now be changing.

But religion has equal positive effects, some through its traditional pastoral role, and some more specific to modern times. In Thailand, for instance, Buddhist monks contribute to the advice network for drug addicts and, as counsellors, are often preferred to medical professionals.

This integration of Western and traditional methods of health care is a key feature of future services in several countries. Neither method can be said to be better than the other, as neither is in itself homogeneous enough to allow a comparison, but elements of both can combine to create the balance of acceptability and effectiveness which is at the heart of satisfactory health care.

The best-known example of a developing country providing a therapeutic lesson for the West comes from India, where support by the extended family is a valuable resource in the long-term management of chronic psychosis. Curiously, that other supposedly family-orientated culture, Italy, is only now awakening to this point as the Italian *famiglia* demands from professional services an equal say in the care of its sick members.

Research and training

Research on health issues is uncommon in most developing countries and research on mental health is even rarer. An International Commission for Health Research and Development has found that 95% of the world's money for health research is spent in the developed world (*Lancet*, 1990). But some countries like Brazil, Mexico and India have made significant efforts to reduce this academic deficit, particularly in those areas most likely to benefit service provision such as estimates of prevalence, aspects of primary care and evaluation of outcome.

Decisions on how best to distribute limited resources are hampered when epidemiological data are lacking and there is no statistical basis for attaching priority to health problems. Sometimes, although it is not ideal, decisions are made according to conspicuous morbidity – you do not have to know how many people have schizophrenia in order to treat those you do know. A less direct short cut is the use of data from neighbouring countries.

Yet in spite of the dearth of information, most countries in this book have estimated needs to the best of their ability and have drawn up national programmes on mental health. The majority of programmes are heavily influenced by the World Health Organization's crusade to develop ample primary care networks in all countries, although mental health professionals have not always found it easy to persuade decision-makers that mental health should be included, as the Chilean experience makes clear.

Training of health personnel is a priority in almost every country included here – the need for suitable personnel, trained to carry out particular health and mental health tasks, is the third common message of transcultural psychiatry. Some countries such as India, Colombia and Thailand already have years of experience in training community health workers. Brazil and Chile, after political disruption of similar training plans, are now gradually regaining lost ground. Libya too is beginning to develop its own programme after years of medical influence by its former colonists and protectors from Western Europe.

Just as most research from developing countries concentrates on the detection and management of psychiatric disorders at a community and primary care level, so training of health personnel focuses on the detection and management of psychiatric problems in primary care. Village health workers, clinic nurses and general practitioners are all seen to be in a position to detect psychiatric disorder, even before it is reported by the person affected, and to treat or refer. Developing countries are clear on the referral pathways which should be followed; Zimbabwe provides an illustration of a two-way chain starting with village workers and ending, several stages later, with specialist hospitals. The UK, with its internal market in which referral may occur sideways across districts according to supply and demand, could learn a lot from such a design.

Developed countries continue to be seen as the best source of postgraduate training by many less developed countries, a reflection not merely of inequality in wealth but of colonial history. But, as Western training institutions themselves come under financial pressure, their courses reflect the demand from doctors in richer countries rather than the public health need of the developing world (Appleby & Araya, 1990).

As with service delivery, the problem is one of centralisation and chaotic referrals. The international system for the delivery of medical education encourages training of the wrong kind and in the wrong place. There is only a rudimentary filter system for controlling how many doctors from individual countries receive postgraduate training in the West, and only recently has there grown a concern over the appropriateness of that training. Some doctors, sponsored by governments or international organisations, receive training in Western medicine or psychiatry which is only partly applicable to care in the developing world. As a result, they remain in the West or return home to set up in private practice.

The introduction of national and regional postgraduate training schemes in the developing world has been one (partial) answer to this. The growth in the West of courses in subspecialties is a better basis for international collaboration.

Health for some?

Despite the varied influence of culture on mental health care, there are also unifying themes between chapters – lack of resources, the fight against stigma, and the need for suitable training. Each of these is worsened by centralised services and poorly defined pathways to care. When psychiatry around the world is described, it therefore teaches two lessons.

The first is the importance of devolving services within countries, towards districts and villages, permitting a rational, clearly delineated system of health care delivery and referral, with prevention, detection and treatment in primary care as its basis. The second is an equivalent devolution of training, suited to primary care and with increasing specialisation tailored to regional or national need, confining referral towards the most sophisticated Western institutions to specific training in subspecialties.

It has become fashionable to acknowledge the importance of culture to mental illness. But culture in this context simply means local need. As such, culture is at the centre of the public health approach to psychiatry with its emphasis on prevention, service delivery to population priorities, and evaluation. And if each of these could be achieved, that genuinely would be a step towards health for all.

References

APPLEBY, L. & ARAYA, R. (1990) Postgraduate training in psychiatry 1977–87: disturbing trends in the pattern of international collaboration. *Medical Education*, **24**, 290–297.

LANCET (1990) Promoting health research for development. *Lancet*, **336**, 1415–1416.

Index

Compiled by STANLEY THORLEY